The Neverending Buzz

Reverse the Aging Process
and Keep Getting Better!

by Tim Farrow

Tim Farrow
Visit my website at www.neverendingbuzz.com

Printed in the United States of America
First Printing: June 2015
Published by Sojourn Publishing, LLC
ISBN: 978-1-62747-125-1
Ebook ISBN: 978-1-62747-126-8
LCN: Pending

This book is dedicated to my parents, my sources of constant inspiration, and to Holly, for all her help in bringing this book into being.

CONTENTS

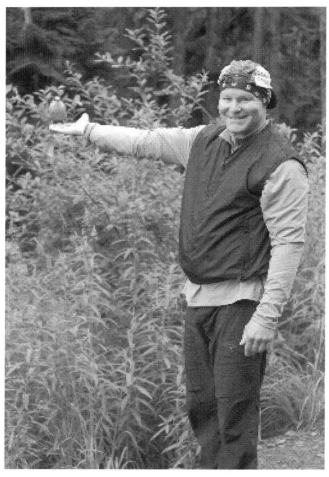

Canada Jay saying hello!

"Obstacles are those frightful things you see when you take your eyes off your goal."

- Henry Ford

INTRODUCTION

I nfinite bliss is your soul's native state. Your body strives to reach and maintain this state over the course of this incarnation. Remove the substances that stand in your way, and you will access happiness such as you have never imagined. In particular, food and drugs, or food as a drug will never give you anything but a temporary sense of gratification that is extremely short-lived.

You can have more of everything as you get older; more energy, more enthusiasm, better sex, more insight, and because you will be more focused on everything you do – more success. You will be more productive at work and at play. Due to this increased productivity, you may be able to retire earlier. You will certainly be able to enjoy your retirement, as few are able to do. For many people, retirement is a state of constant decline. Some retirees can't live full lives simply because there is not enough life left in their body due to years of abuse.

We reach for substances we think will give us some measure of happiness. Instead, these substances erode our quality of life. There is no reason for the body to decline, unless we are trying to find our pleasure in places where it can't be found. We are trying in vain to fill some void. However, you can have real joy that never ends.

You have no idea what your body is capable of achieving. Let me show you what you are missing. If you can summon the will to make a few lifestyle changes, you will be able to access states of happiness you cannot imagine. You can watch as your body transforms before your eyes. You can have fun and joy that few will ever know. As you experience this fun and joy, you bring it into the mass consciousness. As you get more joy out of life, you impart joy to every being on the planet.

We can create whatever we want in this life. The possibilities are endless. We have limited our abilities by reaching for substances that erode our quality of life. As the years go by, these substances take their toll. The toll seems to get steeper as we age. The cost of indulging in these substances becomes greater and greater as we get older. Senescence is the scientific term for physical decline. We experience senescence more and more as the years go by. The body seems to wear out. It is not actually wearing out, but entering into a state of increased dysfunction and pollution.

As we stop this pollution, and start to clean up the mess left behind by substances we thought gave us pleasure, we can reverse the aging process. We can reclaim our youth. Since many of us were not very healthy in our youth, we can experience youth for the first time. These are very bold claims. You may not be inclined to believe me. Good.

Give yourself a chance to experience something you have never imagined. It is much easier than you might think to make changes that give you the happiness you want. We can deconstruct our addictive constructs. We can find freedom. Where do we find freedom? Within, you have it already. You came into this life a free autonomous entity. We accumulated addictions as we went through this life and previous lives. Though these addictions may have been with us for many incarnations, we can drop them in an instant. On the other hand, it may take longer…your choice. When we stop feeding addictions, they cease to live.

Another perk of this lifestyle change – a calm, peaceful feeling unimaginable by anyone who eats a conventional diet. There is much more to gain by cleaning the junk out of your diet than virtually limitless energy, clearer more beautiful skin, and freedom from disease and symptoms of aging.

I'm hoping that somewhere midway through this book, you will become inspired to cleanse from your cabinets and refrigerator all of the junk food that was aging you prematurely and causing you daily consternation. Please throw these foods away rather than giving them to someone, unless you hate them.

I recently had a client who told me I should be proud of her because rather than eating the Christmas cookies she received, she gave them to her neighbor for his children. I asked "oh, did you send them some cigarettes as well?" We see some substances, like soft drinks, high fructose corn syrup, tobacco, etc. as enemies to health. While we demonize these enemies, we may see something like cookies as much more benign. You will soon find out the truth, not by reading this book, but through experiencing the difference ridding yourself of these underappreciated enemies can make to the way you feel and perform. Your adventure awaits.

On the subject of giving junk to children, I know a woman who has been vegetarian for many years but who cooks meat for her son. She doesn't want to make it "off-limits" to him, thereby making him want it even more. She states that he's a "meat and potatoes man". Forbidding children to eat junk food will never work, of course, but that doesn't mean we have to prepare it for them. This is a dilemma every parent who cleans up his or her diet has to wrestle with.

My solution, though I'm not a parent, is to just do what you are doing and influence them by your example. This solution also works when your spouse is not as motivated as you are to make changes. Just do what you are doing and influence them by your example. Never criticize their choices (Good luck with that!). We always want to share the wonderful changes we are experiencing by cleaning our diets and our bodies up. We will help to motivate them much more by carrying on in our own age reversal efforts, and let them witness our positive changes.

The woman I referenced would love her son to eat more healthily. I suggested a bit of positive reinforcement. Her son is a skateboarder. I told her about one of the greatest skateboarders of all time, Bob Burnquist. He is a vegetarian, who at an age when most professional skateboarders would have retired is routinely beating people in competition half his age. Kelly Slater, who at 42 is still on top of his game as the world's most dominant competition surfer. Telling kids about the short-term benefits of a healthy lifestyle, then watching as they start to adopt one, is very gratifying. As with pushing yourself to higher and higher levels, be gentle. Make it fun. What could be more fun than having energy to go on when everyone else has slowed down?

Don't let life pass you by. You can get better with each passing day. You can reverse the damage you have done inadvertently. You can experience peace and tranquility such as you have never imagined. Your skin will become beautiful, soft, and radiant. Your spiritual centers will open up, revealing untapped potential in every area of your life. You can be sexier than you've ever been– even in your youth. You can be more productive at work, and able to retire earlier and in awesome health. Getting rid of the irritants in your diet will dramatically enhance your creativity. Maybe, most importantly, you will become a vector for positive change in this world.

Give cleaning up your diet a good honest try. If you fail, start again. As Yoda said in Star Wars "Do. Or, do not; there is no try" You have nothing to lose but years of accumulated sludge and toxins, as well as your anger.

If we stop eating purely for entertainment, we can have a Buzz that lasts. We can get high and stay high. We can experience life's ups, without the effects of its downs. Rather than eating for temporary sense gratification and boredom relief, we can eat to experience the real bliss. We can attain a state of health unimaginable to most people. Even now, hearing about this, you cannot imagine this state. You have no point of reference. A state of health unsullied by toxic irritants is something you have never experienced—even as a child.

I cannot give you the experience by describing it. It is indescribable anyway. I do invite you to imagine it. Imagine waking up in the morning not groggy and wanting to go back to sleep, but ready to jump up and seize the day. Imagine not having life's little ups and downs have their way with you. Imagine a peace and tranquility at your deepest level that is unaffected by the events of the day. Imagine being able to impart that to everyone you meet through osmosis. Imagine being part of the world solution just by doing what you're doing.

If you can summon the will, if you can love yourself enough to give yourself the gift– right now in the present, the rewards will be beyond your wildest dreams. Endeavoring to imagine a state of perfect health will help you to visualize it and call it in. When you love yourself enough, you cease to limit yourself. This state is who you are; all your aches and pains, your anger, your frustrations, and your limitations have been grafted on to you. You can shake them off anytime you want. Now in this moment, see yourself, as you are – unlimited and absolutely free.

Addiction can have no hold on you unless you choose it. Now is the time to break free. Now is the time to open yourself to limitless possibilities. Limitation is self-inflicted. Declare peace. Relax into super health. Everyone who is successful has an edge. Let this be your edge.

You have the power to make this life anything you want it to be. As you make changes in your life, you empower others by your example. Even those you will never meet will find influence by the changes you make. There is no reason to let our bodies and our planet go into decline because of our addiction. Right now is the time. The present moment is all we will ever have. Youth reclaiming, age reversal, or anything else we choose to call it, is not a future event. It happens right now in the gift of the present.

This book is all about experience. Mine, because I'm sharing with you my experience; and yours because you are about to find out how feeling better than you've ever felt in your life feels. All you have to do is suspend disbelief. No need to believe anything I say. I'm interested in your having the experience. When you have that, you don't need belief. When you have belief, you usually don't get the experience.

In order to age in reverse, you must stop completely all meat, dairy, and wheat. Since eggs are the largest dietary source of cholesterol, they must go too. Soy is not a big part of most people's diets, but I hope to show you how this too qualifies as junk. Fish these days, is so full of toxins that it goes on this list as well. When I refer to junk, crap or other terms of endearment, I am referring to these "foods". A little will be sufficient to keep you on the fast track to old age.

You see, the bad stuff is so much worse than you think. As you clear all this crap from your diet, you will experience a state of health and joy that you have never dreamed. All I ask is that you try it and see for yourself. Age reversal is all about cleaning out the toxins from your diet and your body and replacing the substances that were aging you with substances that will help you feel energized.

I hope to sufficiently inspire you to make these changes. You can feel better in your 50s and 60s than you did in your 20s.

We are often stuck in the thought that we need these substances to be happy. This is not by accident. You have been conditioned to equate happiness and pleasure with these non-foods that are speeding you to decline. It doesn't have to be like that. If you do what you've always done, you'll get what you've always gotten, which is rapid aging, if you're like most everyone else. If you eat what they eat, you will age as they do. Most people are done by the time they are 60; 40 seems to be the cut-off age. You start to notice a drop in vitality by 30, but by 40, you're really feeling it. For one thing, you lose muscle mass. This loss of muscle mass is called sarcopenia and it's a big deal. The average person loses a pound of muscle a year, after age 25. There have been studies that show this is not the case if you strength train. People in their 80s and 90s build muscle if they do some weight training.

I will now share my experience with you. At age 18, I stopped eating meat - just to mess with my mother. Actually, I heard the word "vegetarian" and resonated with the concept of being a non-killer, and as an athlete, I was always looking for an "edge". The next year I backpacked the length of California, on the Pacific Crest Trail. I happened to stop into a health food store at one of my re-supply points, and picked up a book called "Back to Eden," which talked about how bad dairy is for you. I had noticed an unbelievable difference in my energy level and mental clarity because of quitting the meat. Everyone was telling me that I was going to be anemic and not get enough protein. Blah, blah, blah. I immediately realized that dairy must also go.

The difference I felt at 19, from being meat and dairy free was so dramatic, there are no words to describe it. I had so much more energy and endurance than I did before. I felt amazing. The more active you are, the more you notice the changes in diet. I made it my business, when I returned home, to learn more. I read a book called "Become Younger" which talked about how bad meat and dairy are, and added bread to that list. It wasn't widely understood back then just how bad wheat actually is. The early books just talked about how gluten was like glue in your body, and that it would be hard to maintain an ideal weight eating bread and flour products. When I quit eating bread, I felt and enjoyed another dramatic difference. I was finding out how a real "buzz" felt.

I then got the word about raw food and how man is the only animal who cooks his food, how cooking destroys all the life force (living enzymes and probiotics) in the food and how cooking destroys B vitamins and vitamin C. This concept seemed logical. Going mostly raw took me to a completely new level; lotsa fun!

At the same time, I became aware of cleansing. At age 20, I started doing enemas and colonics. In 1976, in Atlanta, there was only one guy offering colonics-$12.00 each. After about my eighth one, I got to the black fecal matter that had been in there a while. I continued to feel better and better through the 80s, as my diet got better and my body got cleaner. I was very much enjoying learning more and experiencing the difference from putting this new knowledge into practice.

In 1997, while doing a dangerous sport called motocross, I dislocated my arm. I knew from experience you don't go outside in Georgia, in August, with a cast on your arm. Once you sweat in a cast, you will itch for the duration. I had broken my collarbone a few years earlier, and put on a bit of fat while convalescing. To avoid putting on fat, I decided to fast for the duration of 3 weeks. Not being able to juice, or do much of anything, I fasted on orange-pineapple juice from a carton, with a little barley-grass powder mixed in. When I got the cast off, and started eating my one raw meal a day (by then I found it best to eat late in the day—like suppertime, and just drink juice during the day). I felt so heavy when I ate again after not eating for 3 weeks. I missed the feeling of lightness I had when I ate only liquid food, so I decided to do smoothies for dinner instead. That was better, but pretty soon the bananas had to go because they were too fibrous. My body seemed to be craving liquid only. Then I tried just juice in the evening - that was what my body wanted. This whole process took only a week or so.

There you have it; my secret is out——no solid food to speak of for 17 years. I don't ever expect to meet another "liquidarian," and certainly don't recommend this to anyone—but it works for me.

I finally had "the big one," a crash to end my motocross career, in 2004. I now have a titanium rod where my left femur is supposed to be. I decided to switch my enthusiasm to bicycling. Motocross is a very intense, whole body workout. I needed an upper-body workout to take motocross's place. I started weight lifting seriously in 2005. I've put on a ton of muscle, all on very little protein. Turns out you don't need much.

Even hard-core body builders are finding out that the body can only absorb about 30 grams of protein at a time. No more are they eating 20 egg whites or a huge steak. It's become the conventional wisdom to instead eat 6-8 small meals a day...some of those meals being liquid (protein shakes). I think that one day it will become conventional wisdom that this is still too much protein, and that keeping your body digesting all day and into the night robs you of energy and vitality.

I should tell you that I'm in it for the high. Nothing tastes as good as feeling good feels. I am sometimes asked something like, "how long are you trying to live?" It's not about that. It's about the buzz. I sometimes tell my life-coaching clients "I wish I could give you one minute to sit in this body and see how this feels." There are no words. I have been so blessed to get the experience early in life. I was not letting anyone tell me I was doing anything wrong. I can honestly say I feel and perform better now—at almost 60, than I did in my 20s, and I was a fit little 20 something. I have not had the experience you are about to have—of reversing the aging process, except that I've gotten fitter and feel more energized as the years go by.

You are about to have the revelation that you have believed something erroneous, something that was killing you slowly. You will find the bad food is so much worse than you thought. As you clean up your diet more and more, you feel the difference. You begin to understand what that stuff was doing to you. When you feel this amazing high, this lightness, this newfound energy, you will not be tempted to stray from your new way of eating and being.

"All things in moderation" is the quote so often cited to justify eating a little crap. Who said that? Ben Franklin. Was he the picture of health? I don't think so. He was a wise and insightful man, but he had that all wrong. Are you going to do a little crack? How about a little crystal meth? Smoke a few cigarettes? Here's a news flash—the bad food is right there with these substances. A little is so much different from none! It doesn't matter what substance you use to erode away your quality of life. If you continue to put junk into the machine, it will continue to run less and less well until it can no longer run at all.

I'd like to clear something up right now. I'm not going to advise you not to smoke, do drugs, or drink soft drinks. I figure if you're reading a book on age reversal you're probably passed that. I'm aiming at an audience motivated to do well by their health. People who could never imagine smoking, drinking soft drinks, or doing drugs but unwittingly erode their health daily with substances that are just as bad. Maybe you have tried some changes and have noticed a difference. If not, hang on to your hat. If so, I hope to motivate you to take it to the next level.

On the subject of smoking and drinking, many people around the world, perhaps you know one, smoke and drink to excess, yet seem healthy. Often the poorest people are the longest lived. It turns out that eating less, even if you still eat a bunch of junk, can be much healthier than what we might consider an adequate diet. Calorie Restriction (CR) is getting a lot of press lately because in any animal species it is tested on CR can increase lifespan.[1] Lots of research now on humans is showing that CR can lower virtually all risk factors for disease and degeneration.

Age reversal will prove to be the most fun you ever had. You may find it easy. A big part of that is thinking it's easy. If you think it will be hard, it will be so. Now my job really begins. It's not enough to tell you of my experience, to give you the facts, as I know them. Not enough to keep you abreast of some of the latest findings and studies. To motivate you, I have to show you how to implement these changes. Actually, I can't really motivate you. Motivation comes from within. I hope you are already motivated and that this book will give you the inspiration to have the experience of reversing the aging process. Easy does it.

Remember, a little of the crap will keep you on the fast track to decline. You must get it all out of your diet in order to age in reverse. You must change your relationship to junk food, to see it for the enemy it is. That part only requires an attitude adjustment. The part where you use freewill to stop and then act is where you may encounter some difficulty. This may bring you face to face with the most common impediment to progress—addiction.

We all fight against addiction to one degree or another. What worked for me was to take the adversarial aspect out of the equation. I'm not fighting. War never works to effect lasting change. I embraced my dark side, thanked it, and moved on. I found that the more of the good stuff I put into my body, the less of the bad stuff I wanted. This is a very profound observation, if I do say so myself. It changed everything. If you find yourself craving some junk food, just eat something good and the craving for the junk will vanish. The more good food we eat the less junk food we crave.

The law of attraction states that what you put your focus on is what you get. If you focus on what you are trying to quit, you will constantly be in battle. If we focus on what we want, we will get what we want! Give yourself the gift of peace, is my advice. Fighting is no fun. Relaxing into a new reality is. I'm all about the fun. When changes are coming fast and easy, it's fun. We yearn for change that is effortless, or as effortless as possible. Take it easy on yourself. Love yourself enough to give yourself the gift of peaceful evolution.

Why are we addicted anyway? It's not your fault. You have been the victim of a relentless attack on your freewill. The media is the worst offender here. Your samskaras,[2] or past life tendencies, may also play a role. Don't worry, this can all change in an instant, or it may take longer, your choice. Remember, it's very unnatural to eat dead, decaying flesh. Another animal's milk, or even that from our own species as an adult, is not your native food. Likewise, synthetic starch, GMO food like corn and soy is also not what our bodies want, which means this kind of food is easy to walk away from. Don't let your conditioning keep you from finding out what's possible with these wonderful bodies. Your body will guide you to the next level– and the next. As you clean up your act, its voice will get louder. Listen.

Everywhere we look, we are bombarded with advertising aimed at our need for happiness and fulfillment. The most blatant must surely be "open happiness." There are so many more. Some I've seen recently include "help yourself to happiness"—Golden Corral. "Live mas" (more) Taco Bell. "Unwrap paradise"—Almond Joy. I recently saw a commercial for a ready to bake cookie dough that had the slogan "bake some love". This list could go on and on; Even if you reject this sort of mental invasion intellectually, it gets in subliminally.

These people are good at what they do. Whatever we do in this life, we choose because we think it will make us happy. If someone holds something up and says, "This will make you happy," you have to listen. At least your subconscious does. Making you equate junk food with love is pure marketing genius. Again, your subconscious is very susceptible to this sort of programming, especially when you see these messages played repeatedly in many different forms.

Then there's the perceived peer pressure. This is largely illusionary. I've found it really doesn't detract from social interaction not to eat what someone else is eating. We sometimes feel that it puts some sort of wall up between us when we don't validate someone else's choice by doing the same thing they're doing. Actually, you're doing them a service no one else may ever do them. Showing them a new way of being. I've found when I sit down with someone and do not have what they're having, it starts a conversation something like "don't you like this?" I explain that it's not a matter of taste. I'm doing something different. It is about nourishing my body not about indulging my addictions. The way my body feels makes up for any temporary sense gratification I may be missing. I am eating for a different reason than they are. No one in their whole life has ever showed them this approach.

A social interaction that is centered on food is a perfect time to share your newfound way of eating and consequent zest for life. Bring a dish to share with everyone. Chances are very good they will like what you brought better than what else is being served. Healthy food can taste better than junk food. All it takes is a little creativity and a bit of education. There are many books out there on how to prepare healthy food. Even raw foods can be unbelievably tasty.

When we crave a food, what is it we want? Taste. We think that we may derive a bit of pleasure from the temporary gratification this indulgence may bring. We crave a drug effect. Like drugs, food promises much, but delivers so little. Think about it, if you do a drug or have a drink, you're feeling the effect for a while, several hours usually. Eat some junk; you get the buzz of taste for a few minutes. Not much bang for the buck, so little pleasure for so much damage.

I often hear people say something like "I'd like to have a better diet, but I just love cheesecake." For me it was ice cream. We all have something we love but would love to quit. Why do we love it? Because we say we love it. We create the reality for ourselves by using a powerful word like "love" in connection with something we are trying to quit. In other words, you love it because you have decided to love it. It's no good pushing what you don't want away, because that focuses your mental energy on that which you don't want. All you have to do is stop saying you love it. We are such powerful creators. Time to start creating what you want.

You can have a buzz that lasts. Feeling good physically is the best high there is. Trust me; I've done many different ones. If you could feel what this is about, you would kill for this buzz. No killing will be required though. You don't even have to kill your addiction; just stop feeding it. Yes, sometimes you may be weak and give in to your old habits. No worries, just start again. The longer you go between binges, the more you will feel the adverse effect when you do cave. Then you will be stronger the next time, remembering what it felt like when you ate that do-do. You will start to see more and more clearly, what this stuff is. It is not pleasure but pain. It is slow death and fast decline.

Remember, the vast majority eats this crap on a daily basis. They are also getting old fast. If you want something different, you will have to do something different. The difference is so dramatic that you will not be tempted to eat junk when you feel the new buzz. Nothing tastes as good as feeling good feels. Why would you trade the most wonderful feeling you ever felt for some crap food?

Willpower is only needed to make the initial change. Once you turn the corner, you will not be tempted. It's like driving a car. You're going down the road in a straight line—very little effort needed. When a turn comes up, it's another matter. Now you must brake and make some calculations. You must turn the wheel and make the change in direction. Once you start down the next straight, you can relax and enjoy the ride. That's what you will find when you change your diet. It may be hard at first, but stay with it. It gets easier and easier. Now you're cruising to the Promised Land. Who promises it? I do. I'm there. Nothing is stopping you but you.

You will find age reversal applies to all facets of your life. You will heal from injury so much faster than before. Remember when you were young how you used to bounce back from injury? You will also not sustain injury as easily as you did when you weakened your body by eating all that crap. Also, you will feel like moving. When you ate junk, you felt weak and tired. Now you feel like you gotta do something.

This energy is not a giddy, "can't sit still" kind of thing. It's just there, on tap. Actually, you will feel calmer than you've ever felt in your life.

Let's say you had some accident and had an injury to your neck. If those muscles are strong, you will be able to shrug it off and maybe be a little sore for a day or two. If you have less muscle in your neck, you may well break something. Speaking of necks, that is one of the first places people show their age. How many folks do you know with a "wattle," or sagging neckline? The jowls sag and fill with fat. Not a pretty picture, especially when you remember what they used to look like. Look at aging TV or music stars. How fast some of them age, and how others seem to do much better.

This is not genetic. It's lifestyle. Genetics doesn't take you very far if you continue to wage war on your body by filling it full of toxins. On the other hand, someone very close to me has defied his genetics—my dad. Both of his parents died of heart disease, his father died at 46. His brother is long gone. He, at 84 is still kickin' it. He does some exercise every day. He's almost vegetarian. I'm hoping this book will inspire him to completely give up the soy, wheat, and dairy.

My writing guru, Tom Bird, tombird.com, had his biological age determined by his doctor. By the way, if you have aspirations of writing a book and lack the motivation or the confidence to do so, this guy can help you. The doctor determined his biological age to be 26. He is 57, but by virtue of 22 years being vegetarian, 13 being vegan, and his generally healthy lifestyle, which includes yoga and light exercise every day, his doctor says he has the body of a 26-year-old.

So now, I'm wondering. Since I'm almost 60, have been vegetarian for 41 years, vegan for 40, what must my biological age be? Maybe 19? Actually, I feel better now than I did when I was 19. I was a super fit 19-year-old, turning 20 somewhere in California, backpacking the length of the state on the Pacific Crest Trail. I am more fit now and feel so much better than I did at 19. For instance, three months ago I rode the highest lift-served downhill mountain bike trail on Whistler Mountain, British Columbia. The trail's name is, "Top of the World," and starts at the very top of the mountain. Definitely, the rockiest, steepest bit of riding I've ever done. Very few people ride this trail.

Last month, I rode my bicycle 201 miles in just under 17 hours. That is, by far, the longest I've ever ridden. I couldn't do that when I was 19! I'm not recommending you ride like that—it hurts your butt. I'm not advocating my liquid diet for anyone else either. I AM hoping you get to experience aging in reverse.

This month, I rode several trails in Moab, Utah. These trails were a lot rockier and rougher than I expected. My riding partner on this trip was 21 years younger than me. We did a shuttle run to the top of a trail called "The Whole Enchilada." I took a very hard trip over the handlebars. This type of fall is known as an Endo. I slammed really hard onto rock, severely bruising both my thighs, and causing my left elbow quite a bit of trauma as well. I can't say I got up immediately, but when I did, I remounted and finished the ride. We had several hours left to go. I was in quite a bit of pain the rest of the ride. Most 60-year-olds would not have been on that trail in the first place. They certainly would not have gotten up from a fall like that and been able to continue. The benefits of reversing your age go way beyond just feeling better and looking younger. You can keep bouncing back from injury the way you did when you were younger.

I hope to communicate to you the joy that reversing your age brings. I hope to help you understand just how insidious many of the foods people enjoy every day are to your health. I hope to inspire you to make these changes yourself. It can be hard, but it need not be. Just take it easy on yourself, enjoy the process, and relax. We must strike a balance between pushing ourselves to the next level, and enjoying the level we are on. We must be gentle, yet keep striving to be better. This is not about longevity for me, I will say again. The feeling of being in a youthful body that will support anything you want to do, defies description. Getting rid of the bad food is essential to get you there. You may do it quickly or it may be a process. Relax into it, in whatever form it takes.

You could say that age reversal is a three-stage process whereby you first slow aging down by eating less of the foods that cause aging and supplementing some nutrients you may not be getting enough of. Stopping the aging process may be the next step. You will attain this step when you stop these foods completely. Remember these foods are meat, fish, dairy, eggs, wheat, and soy. The other part of reaching this step is eating a lot more of the foods that build your health. These include vegetables, fruit, beans, nuts, seeds, seaweed, onions, mushrooms, and lots of salad. When you have sufficiently cleansed the toxins you already have from the body, age reversal can truly start. I hope to teach you how to do this.

Think of yourself in transition. This transition can be as quick or as slow as you desire. Your addictions will conspire to keep you where you are. Don't let them. Once you understand why you are addicted, and have started to wriggle out from under addiction's grasp, you will start to accelerate in the process. To start your transition, I recommend learning a new way to breathe which will connect you to your unlimited nature and loosen addictions hold on you.

Breathing is very important because oxygen is what we live on. You can go for weeks or months without food and days or weeks without water. Without oxygen, unless you are an advanced yogi or seasoned free diver, you will die within 3 to 5 minutes. Also in the air is prana or chi. Prana[3] is the life force energy that is all around us. As we breathe it in, this life force gives us life. Most people do not breathe very well. They breathe shallowly and quickly. The average person breathes upwards of 20 times a minute. Some advanced yogis breathe once or twice a minute, yet get more oxygen and life force than the average person. How?

Actually, it's all in the exhale. Our lungs have four lobes, or chambers; two upper, and two lower. Most people don't really engage the lower lobes because they breathe with the chest only. Observe your breathing right now. Your chest is probably rising and falling at least a little. What we want to do is bring the breath deeper into the body. We want to engage the lower lobes. Watch a baby breathe. The chest stays still. The belly expands and contracts. This is what we want to achieve. We want to reconnect with the natural way to breathe.

So here it is. Exhale all the way out; contract the abdomen. Pull the belly button in as far as you can. Deflate the balloon as it were. Push the breath out forcefully yet gently. You can always exhale more. As you get to the bottom of the exhale, experiment with blowing out even more. Use your abdominal muscles to draw the belly in as you would if you were having your picture taken or met a hot member of the opposite sex. (Or the same sex—gotta be politically correct) This also massages the abdominal organs, stimulating movement in the lower GI tract. It's even a light ab workout.

Here is a good trick to know when you leave a building that has toxins from new carpet, paint, or cigarette smoke. When you get outside exhale completely and then force the breath out with several short further exhalations, making a sound like huh, huh, huh. If you've been in a smoky environment, you might even see smoke come out your mouth.

We hear about how we should be breathing from our diaphragms. Many yoga teachers and sports coaches talk about this—bringing the breath deeper into the body for more complete oxygenation. The diaphragm however, is an involuntary muscle, so it's hard to connect with it. It's hard to visualize what this muscle is doing. The breathing technique I'm sharing with you connects you with the diaphragm. The diaphragm has no nerve endings, and so cannot be felt. When you use this abdominal breath technique, you are engaging the diaphragm.

When you exhale, you release tension throughout your whole body. When you inhale, tension increases. The good news is we don't really have to inhale. All we have to do is allow the new breath. We are "negative pressure" breathers, which means when you exhale a vacuum is created in your lungs. Air will always rush in to fill a vacuum if it can. This is why you can't kill yourself by holding your breath. You will just pass out and start breathing again. So on the inhale expand the abdomen, making the Buddha belly. Inflating the balloon.

If you practice sucking the belly in on the exhale and pushing it out on the inhale, this will soon become your natural way of breathing. What this will mean is that you are getting more oxygen into the body with every breath. This will also slow down the rate of respiration. You will be breathing less times a minute. This slower, longer rate of respiration slows down the heart. Breath drives the heart, not vice versa. Since the heart only gets to rest between beats even when you're asleep, this is very significant. Giving the heart some rest is definitely a good thing.

Breathing this way makes you calm and peaceful; the opposite way that people breathe when they feel nervous, angry, or agitated. When you are mad, you breathe shallowly and quickly. Funny how in the English language mad can also mean insane. Instead of getting angry, if you remember to breathe, you may not have to go temporarily insane. As Eckhart Tolle says in his excellent book "A New Earth," "it's never about what happens." Meaning…we don't have to be controlled by circumstance. We don't have to be the victim of what happens.

Many people are drawn to the idea of meditation. They may try it without much success, even if someone instructs them on how to do it. Meditation has all sorts of health benefits, from lowering blood pressure to calming brain waves and heart rhythm. Meditation has even been shown to enhance immune system function. Meditation is a state of non-thinking. It's been said, "Meditation is not what you think." To sit or lay down and not think is extremely hard for most of us. If you sit quietly and do this abdominal breathing technique for a few minutes, you will almost be there. Then all you have to do is put the focus at the third eye; the point between your eyebrows, and watch the movie. Make sure you do not clench your jaw. If you watch long enough you'll get a blank screen, with perhaps a point of light or several points of light on it. Keep breathing and watch that point of light. See what happens.

Breathing this way also connects you to your heart center—your intuitive center. Most of us live in our heads. When you are guided only by the brain, you are easily confused. You could say the heart, the intuitive voice within, is the voice of God. The heart is never confused or undecided. Tune into its guidance through this breath technique. The heart is completely free of addictions. The more you connect with it, the less old thought forms will sway you.

I'm not implying that you have to meditate in order to age in reverse. Meditation is an excellent tool to help you gain control of yourself. The Masters tell us God is within us. All we need to do is open ourselves to the light and the darkness vanishes. There may seem to be a lot of darkness around now in the form of fear, but the light is much more powerful. Connect with your unlimited soul in any way that works for you. I like to connect with mine by bouncing down the side of a mountain on my bicycle.

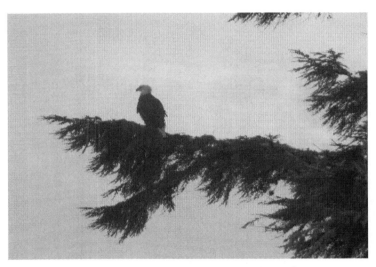

Bald Eagle in Clayoquot Sound, Tofino

"Conformity is the jailer of freedom and the enemy of growth."

\- John F. Kennedy

CHAPTER 1
DOCTORS DUEL—YOU WIN

Doctors used to be thought of as the antithesis of nutritional knowledge. My brother graduated from medical school a few years ago. I asked him about what they teach on nutrition these days. He said they tell you it's good to have a balanced diet but that it doesn't cure or cause disease. This means doctors are largely oblivious to the cause and effect of diet.

Some doctors are educating themselves. This is still the exception rather than the norm, but is a very encouraging development. Those who are learning about diet and its role in making or breaking our health, often focus on one or more areas of diet science. Sometimes, they seem not to get the bigger picture. For instance, Dr. William Davis wrote a groundbreaking book called "Wheat Belly". While giving us vital information about how wheat is destroying our health, at the same time, he advocates eating meat and even dairy, another book called, "Grain Brain" by Dr. David Perlmutter follows a similar course.

These authors have furthered the cause of super health to a huge degree because wheat attacks your health in so many ways. The problem is they trade one evil for another. No worries. We don't have to go with everything they say. We can learn a lot from what they have to tell us about the evils of wheat, without swallowing their message whole. Likewise, Kaayla T. Daniel, Ph.D. in her excellent book "The Whole Soy Story" gives us a heads up about how horrible soy consumption is to our health. She also recommends meat as a healthy food.

This book is extremely informative and comprehensive on the dangers of soy. I recommend these books highly. Just be aware that if you eat meat you will continue to age at an accelerated rate. You will be filling your arteries with plaque, and consuming huge amounts of antibiotics, growth hormone, and pesticides.

In the other corner, we have doctors such as Dr. Caldwell B. Esselstyn, whose book "Prevent and Reverse Heart Disease" tells us how Bill Clinton, after a heart scare, took up a vegan diet and improved his health dramatically. Dr. Neil Barnard in his book "Protect Your Brain" tells us that occluded arteries cause Alzheimer's, dementia and stroke. He advises us to stop eating animal products to reverse this damage. He recommends "healthy whole grains" as part of a diet that omits all animal foods. If we read "Wheat Belly," we know most whole grains are anything but healthy.

Dr. Joel Fuhrman in his book "Eat to Live" actually calls Dr. Davis out for his advice to eat meat. He calls meat eating extremely unhealthy. He is also not buying the fact that wheat causes so many problems. You see now why so many people are confused. Dr. Fuhrman in his book "The End of Dieting" tells us to lose weight we need not count calories. All we need to do is follow his "nutraterian" (nutrient dense) way of eating. He goes with my idea of putting more of the good stuff in and watching the desire for the crap fall away. He wants you to eat a lot of salad, and is a big believer in beans as a healthy food. He says as long as you omit certain types of food. You need not count calories. I love his quote "moderation kills." In other words, if you try to include foods that attack your health in small amounts, you still do damage, and will not attain your health goals. Small amounts are certainly better than large amounts, but the magic happens when you completely stop eating the foods that age you.

Dr. Fuhrman says our LDL cholesterol should not be over 100. In preparation for this book, I decided to have mine checked. My number? 126. How could I be over the optimal number?! Maybe, it's the red palm oil I go out of my way to consume. Dr. Fuhrman states palm oil and coconut oil are the only saturated fats in the vegetable kingdom. I read elsewhere that while this was true, it didn't really matter. Maybe it does. I am certainly now going to experiment with eliminating red palm oil, and see what happens.

I have used coconut oil as a moisturizer for my entire body for many years, and will continue to do so. Many people use it for cooking because it has a low flashpoint; in other words, high temperatures do not harm coconut oil. Maybe this is a bad idea. Maybe saturated fat of any kind is a bad thing. Since I don't cook, I have never used coconut oil for anything other than a topical moisturizer or sexual lubricant. Try the coconut oil as a moisturizer to seal in cellular water and lubricate the skin, allowing it to stay supple and young looking.

Dr. Robert Huizenga, of TVs "Biggest Loser" fame, says that counting calories is essential to success in weight loss and that you should keep calorie intake well under 2000 a day. He wants you to exercise a minimum of 90 minutes a day. This approach has resulted in huge sustainable weight loss in many people. It has also gotten many off prescription drugs; lowering blood pressure, cholesterol numbers, fasting glucose, homocysteine, and many other disease predictors. He says people who use the excuse of not having enough time to exercise would make the time if they realized how important exercise actually is. He says if you had cancer, you would FIND time to try to cure it. His program can cure cancer before it starts.

Gary Null Ph.D., who has been on the scene for many years, is firmly in the camp of the vegan leaning doctors. This

3

guy must be somewhere around 70 years old. I saw him on PBS recently doing a talk and promoting his latest book. Judging by the way that he looks, I would say he's on to something. He advocates no meat, dairy, fish, or eggs. He does however, seem to be missing the soy message. You would think a person as well informed as he is would have heard by now how bad soy is for you. Maybe he's just not buying it.

Dr. Howard Murad, whose book "The Water Secret" alerts us to the dangers of not getting enough cellular water. He tells us salt is the enemy of cellular water. He states for every gram of salt consumed, it takes 23 grams of cellular water to eliminate it. Cellular water, he says, is not replenished by simply drinking water. Cellular water can become permanently depleted, and is a cause of aging. He advises us to eat our water, as water contained in plants is the kind that replenishes our cellular water. Fresh fruit and vegetable juice also replenishes cellular water. Loss of cellular water is at the heart of many aging systems. This is a huge reason why skin sags and wrinkles. He is another doctor who recommends a plant-based diet.

Dr. Stephen Masley has a very interesting book called "Thirty Days to a Younger Heart." He actually uses the term age reversal. He calls it "turning back the clock on aging." Dr. Masley has some unique points to make. He offers a demonstration of what consumption of dairy does to your arteries. He pours a glass of whole milk, then pours the glass back into a pitcher, and holds the glass up. You see a film of fat around the inside of the glass. This is showing the sticky nature of butterfat, the kind that's in milk and dairy products. This type of fat is one of the worst fats for clogging arteries. He helps us understand the nature of plaque accumulation in our arteries. I thought as most people do that heart attacks are caused by arteries that become first 50% blocked then 60%, then 70% and so on. He states most heart attacks happen because arterial plaque that may not be that thick dislodges and migrates to an area that also has occlusion, causing complete blockage to the artery. He agrees with Dr. Fuhrman that beans are one of nature's perfect foods.

Dr. Masley has some other interesting observations to share with us. He says that for every woman who dies of breast cancer, six die of heart disease. (I've read elsewhere that the figure is as high as ten) Half the people who die of heart disease have "normal" cholesterol. He also says that fully 50% of people over 55 have metabolic syndrome, which we will discuss later in our discourse about wheat, which has been shown to almost single-handedly cause this new epidemic. The ADA (American diabetes Association) puts this number much higher.

He is a huge believer in magnesium, citing the many problems caused by magnesium deficiency. Dr. Masley tells us calcium supplementation can wipe out our stores of magnesium. When we have too much calcium in the body, magnesium is depleted. He says everyone should take a magnesium supplement daily and that usually calcium supplementation does more harm than good. Masley also states Magnesium Malate and Magnesium Glycenate are the types best assimilated by the body. Magnesium Citrate is okay, but not as good. He says Magnesium Oxide is the one you want to avoid.

It has long been known that Magnesium deficiency causes muscle cramps. Many people have problems with cramps. Athletes can be effected by muscle cramping, especially if those muscles haven't been used in a while or if they are really trying to push the envelope.

He states that one meal containing the wrong kind of fat (saturated– animal origin) constricts arteries by 20% for six hours after the meal. This is why so many people die of heart attacks soon after eating.

I love Dr. Masley's quote "breakfast is the most important meal of the day – to drink." He wants us to have a big smoothie with lots of fruit or vegetables, and some flax thrown in for breakfast. We will talk about this in depth in a later chapter.

Dr. Furhman makes the point that if our diets contain enough calories to get us through the day, we automatically get enough protein. He asks us "which do you think has more protein calorie for calorie, broccoli, or beefsteak?" Answer? Broccoli. He alerts us to the dangers of too much protein. This is not new knowledge. Too much protein causes a huge array of health problems, more on this later.

Dr. Furhman tells us olive oil has too many calories to be used on a daily basis for most people. I had never heard this before. One thing he said that positively blew me away is that you could drink water from the Great Lakes for 100 years and not get the concentration of toxins you would get from eating 1 pound of fish from those lakes. He recommends you eat no more than two servings of fish a week, and preferably don't eat it more than once a month. Say what, Doc? Shouldn't that read, "avoid fish like the plague?" I know he's trying to make his diet doable for people, but if fish is that poisonous, and he would never eat it, why not advise people to leave it alone entirely? Even so, I consider his book "Eat to Live" a must read for anyone interested in attaining super health.

I read an interview in Life Extension Magazine with Dr. Donald Schnell. He has co-authored a book with Marilyn Diamond, author of the bestseller "Fit for Life". They have a whole chapter on vitamin D deficiency. He has this to say, "For nearly 30 years a collective group of individuals from the dermatology associations, governmental regulatory agencies, and the media have been on a campaign to prevent healthy and safe sun exposure. What they want you to ignore is a historical fact. We've had a positive relationship with the sun for as long as humanity has been on the planet. What you're not told is that scores of respectable researchers, epidemiologists, and dermatologists have published studies that show that sunlight is good for your health."

He tells us that men with low vitamin D levels suffered over twice as many heart attacks. He laments the fact that millions of dollars are spent advertising cholesterol-lowering drugs, but vitamin D supplementation is universally overlooked.

Dr. Schnell has this to say about vitamin C "Every time you consume vitamin C, somewhere in your body you stop aging. Somewhere you stimulate repair. Somewhere you bring about detoxification. Somewhere you eradicate infection and prevent free radical damage. Somewhere your skin will clear up. You may see fewer wrinkles on your face. According to an article in the August 2002 issue of Biological Psychiatry, you'll have more sex and less depression, and you'll ward off serious disease. And, all this is just scratching the surface, because vitamin C is a miraculous healing nutrient."

We can add him to the list of vegan leaning doctors. I have not read his book called "Young for Life." Sounds like a good one. He also has a lot to say about sarcopenia – the muscle wasting that occurs as we age. He says with less muscle your metabolism slows down and when it does you, burn less calories and have less energy. He calls this downward spiral "Sedentary Death Syndrome." Indeed, we have heard from many voices in many different ways—the only reason our metabolism slows down is sarcopenia – muscle atrophy.

What can we learn from all of these doctors and their many approaches to optimizing our health? One thing is that we need not believe everything anybody says. We must test everything for ourselves. In this book, I am endeavoring to help you understand just how insidious meat, fish, dairy, eggs, wheat, and soy really are. This may seem radical, but it is really just bringing all these doctor's messages together. You can make up your own mind about calorie counting. I go more with Dr. Furhman, hoping you end up eating a lot more salads, vegetables, beans, fruits, nuts and seeds. He states that you need not worry about calories if you're eating these foods almost exclusively. He allows meat and dairy in tiny amounts as condiments. I disagree with this. I intend to show you just how bad these substances are, and how eating any is a serious insult to your health.

I must include in this discussion Dr. D'Adamo's widely influential book "Eat for Your Type." He states Type O blood is the original blood type from which the other types evolved, which is why it's the universal donor type. He says people with Type O blood are generally more robust and tend to live longer. He states people with Type O blood need to eat at least some meat, but that people with Type A, B and AB blood should avoid meat at all costs. No other health expert I know of shares his opinion. Nevertheless, his book has had quite an impact. People with Type O blood may very well handle meat and other toxins better than people with Type A, B or AB, but they will suffer earlier decline and a greater danger of heart disease and cancer if they heed his advice.

Before we leave this little discourse on the many approaches to optimizing your health, I would like to make note of one more author. John Robbins, heir to the Baskin-Robbins Ice Cream fortune, wrote a book in the 80s called "Diet for a New America." This was the first book I read that really elucidated the environmental destruction caused by our meat and dairy addictions. I recommend this book to everyone. I hope you will read some of the books that I've mentioned, especially this one. He was disinherited because he wrote this book. His family threatened he would not receive a dime of inheritance if this book was published. Since he lost his inheritance to educate us, help a brother out – buy his book. Just kidding, it was a bestseller.

So what, if anything do these doctors agree on? In a word, vegetables. Vegetables should form the basis of any healthy diet. Lettuce and green leafy vegetables are probably the healthiest foods known to man. As you drop the foods from your diet that were hastening your demise, you will have room for lots of vegetables. Finding new ways of preparing these will be part of your new adventure into the wonderful world of age reversal.

You see, what I am advocating as to the foods we must stop eating in order to age in reverse is not that radical. I am bringing together the best all these doctors have to teach us. Some have major blind spots, and focus on only one aspect of dietary health. The approach I am bringing you considers many new findings that are bearing out what I have experienced. Getting rid of the insidious "foods" that are destroying our health is the greatest gift you can give yourself.

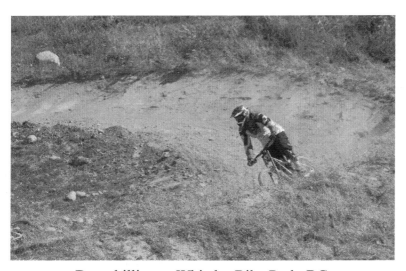

Downhilling at Whistler Bike Park, BC

"If at first, the idea is not absurd then there is no hope for it."

\- Albert Einstein

CHAPTER 2
EXTREME? WHO'S EXTREME?

Maybe I should ask whose extreme? I submit that if anyone should be considered extreme it would be those who eat whatever they want thinking it is bringing them some measure of happiness, thinking the joy that is lacking in their lives can be found in some substance be it food or drug, or food as drug. I consider it extreme to go through life like a child, with minimal self-control; no willpower to do anything other than what their addictions and the media dictate to them. When you have a nation of other adult-children, then someone who actually has some measure of free will looks extreme.

I read something years ago, I can't remember where, wherein the author was observing how most adults have not attained much emotional maturity. In other words though they're in adult bodies (which are aging rapidly) they act like children. Since I read that, I have begun to observe this too. Look how people drive. "No you're not getting in front of me". Look at our political climate. "My bombs are more powerful than yours". When it comes to food choices, most of us are as powerless as little kids at doing what we know is optimal, especially when all the other little kids who are compelled reinforce this behavior by indulging their addictions. Then you have the media run by a bunch of greedy little kids......... You get the idea. Seeing others in this light gives you compassion for them. I'm not saying I'm not a child too. I like to think I'm a child in a different way than most people. Maybe that's just the kid in me talking.

People, who would label us extreme because we make healthy food choices, have no idea what this lifestyle is about. They have no idea how our bodies feel, and how the desire for the crap food has left us long ago. We know where they are. We've been there. They have no idea where we are. It is our joy to show them. Actions speak louder than words. By showing them a new way of being, we help to hasten their evolution just by doing what we're doing. Never think you can't make a difference. By doing age reversal you are helping everyone on the planet to evolve, to mature.

Back when I became vegetarian, the word meant somebody who only eats vegetable matter. The word "vegan" was not even coined yet. I never did really like that word, it sounds kind of wimpy. Before "vegan" came along, if you were a vegetarian who still ate dairy they called you "lactovegetarian", if you ate eggs too it was "ovo lactovegetarian", if you ate fish it was "pisceterian". Don't ask me where that word came from. I recommend we call vegetarians who still do dairy "mucovegiterians", eggs, "cholesterterians", and fish, "toxiterians". Just messing around. Who cares what anybody calls anybody? If somebody calls you extreme, take it as a compliment. You're not doing what they are doing. You're not aging at the rate they are aging. You are aging in reverse.

If either eating the junk that everybody eats, and taking the drugs they take to compensate for their unhealthy habits, or to try to put some joy into their lives is normal, I'm happy to be called extreme or radical or restrictive. Actually, I see them as restrictive. They restrict how much fun they can have and how good they can feel in their later years, and indeed in their present years. We know about their craziness. They don't know about our craziness. We have something the vast majority of people will never have.

The more of us that do this age reversal thing, the more of us that will. What I mean is the mass consciousness is a very real phenomenon. We are all connected. We all influence each other. As you do age reversal, you become an influencer instead of one of the influenced! As our free will develops and awakens, we cease to be influenced by the mass consciousness and we start to do the influencing. If you ever wanted to "save the planet", this is the way. Humanity is in trouble. We are at a crossroads. The direction we take will be dictated by the individual choices each of us makes. As you do age reversal, you become part of the solution.

Drugs are substances we use to compensate for something that is missing or not working in our lives and our bodies. If there are disease systems, or something we want to get rid of in the body, like cholesterol, we hope a drug can help us rid ourselves of it. Likewise, when something is missing in our lives, we hope a drug can give us something to fill the void. When we are in pain, either physical or emotional, we reach for our drug of choice to dull the pain and give us something to feel. Alcohol is effective in this regard, as it is a numbing agent.

For many of us our drug of choice is food. I call it the Food As Drug (FAD) syndrome. You've heard of fad diets. This FAD diet never goes out of fashion. Just about all of us are food addicts. We don't realize we are addicted until we try to quit some type of food. To age in reverse we must quit several types of food. However, unlike addicts of other drugs, we do not have to simply quit. We are able to replace. Replacing is much easier than quitting. All we have to do is start eating more of the truly healthy foods. When we do, the desire for the junk food falls away on its own.

The addictive thought forms however, are very strong. As long as they are fed, they will continue to hold sway in your life. An alcoholic, once he has made up his mind to be sober, can never drink again. Even a small amount will feed the addictive behavior. Likewise, a small amount of the food you are trying to avoid will keep the addiction going. In addition, a small amount of the food that is aging you at an accelerated rate is going to keep doing so. These are reasons why a little is so different from none.

We throw up many blocks for ourselves. Rather I should say our addictive thought forms throw up many blocks to freedom. One of my good friends feels he needs to eat something like chicken or fish when he takes his clients out to lunch. This is the way he keeps himself addicted. He is also laboring under the delusion that chicken and fish are better for him than beef. He quit red meat years ago, but will never be able to reverse the aging process, or even achieve optimal health while his meat addiction is being fed. I asked him if, being the owner of his company, he hadn't reached a station in life where he didn't have to kowtow to someone else's perceived expectations. I doubt his clients would care if he had a salad while they had a steak. The quote "If you knew how little people notice what you do, you wouldn't worry that they will" comes to mind. I think we have all reached a station in life where we don't have to worry about what anyone else might think of us. It's time to let go of the fear and embrace true self-love.

If you want to stay in your comfort zone, that's your choice—and a popular choice it is. Like the "comfort foods" that make us decidedly uncomfortable, the comfort zone is largely illusionary. If you want to stay the same, I respect your wish. This wish cannot be granted however. Nothing in the physical universe is static. Everything either progresses or regresses. Nothing stays the same. You decide where you go from here. You call the shots—until you run out of bullets.

I can't relate to non-progression. I feel the need to expand my awareness, to make more and more sense of this illusion we call life, to progress in the eternal now. The gift is the present. This moment is all we'll ever have. I also feel the need for speed. I enjoy changes that come fast and joyfully. I choose to make progression fun and easy. Staying the same is not an option. Why would anyone want to stay the same? There is so much more to experience and to feel if we open ourselves to new ways of thinking—and being.

Paramahansa Yogananda said, "People are so skillful in their ignorance". We have many ways of deluding ourselves. We must be ever vigilant in the beginning of our quest for freedom, that these old thought forms do not continually sabotage our efforts. The media and the mass consciousness we are all tapped into to some degree also conspire to keep us stuck. Once you get a taste of true freedom, once your free will begins to call the shots, you will no longer be under the power of any external force. Your old thought forms trying to reestablish themselves will never fool you.

Eckhart Tolle, in his book "A New Earth", states that the ego is always trying to keep you where you are—under its spell, because it senses its own demise at the end of this incarnation. It feels threatened and wants to preserve itself. Likewise, your addictive thought forms seem to want to keep you where you are, but like the ego they are all part of this illusion we call life. The fact that it is an illusion means you can make any change in it you want! This is how the spiritual Masters perform their so-called miracles. We are all spiritual Masters who haven't realized it yet. The value of a book like "A New Earth" is that once you understand how the ego operates in you, you can spot it at work and claim freedom from it. Once you begin to recognize all the myriad ways your addictive thought forms attempt to assert themselves, you are on the road to true freedom. May your road be short and easy.

Finding the freedom within to reverse the aging process and feeling the difference will be the greatest blessing in your life. If you find it hard in the beginning, analyze your thoughts. You will begin to see through all the many masks addiction wears. You'll begin to see the messages the media and the mass consciousness sends us in a new light. You'll begin to laugh at the absurdity of it all. You will begin to see life as a great entertaining play that you can watch but not be affected by. Maybe I'm getting too esoteric here, but the blessing of soul freedom goes way beyond establishing free will.

The old saying, "success breeds success, failure breeds failure" applies here. As you find success in establishing your free will where food choices are concerned, this success will spill over into every facet of your life. You will increase your willpower by using it. That willpower will then be available in ever-greater amounts to help you achieve any goal you set your mind to. As you get used to calling the shots for yourself– unaffected by past conditioning, you will be able to access greater and greater measures self-control and power. You will be able to push past old limitations in every part of your life.

There are no words to describe the difference between being free and being stuck in old thought forms. One definition of "belief" is a recurring thought form. Again, there is no need for belief when you have experience. One benefit of finding real freedom is the calm peaceful feeling you get from not consuming the caustic irritants that form such a large part of most people's regimens.

Salt is one of those irritants. Runners often get chafing between their legs or under their arms, because of skin on skin friction. I noticed that once I quit the salt, this was a thing of the past for me. Anything that irritates the outside irritates the inside as well. If you stop consuming this particular irritant for a while, and then consume salt either on purpose or in something, you will find the food you have it in tastes horrible. Salt is an acquired taste that your body loses taste for very quickly. As your body and your taste buds "wake up", you will find you have lost the taste for many of the substances you used to enjoy. This goes especially for any type of recreational drug you might have used. Once you feel good, any artificial high you might experience just takes you out of your natural buzz. I guarantee nothing artificial can compare to the way super health feels.

Take my word for it............no don't! Experience for yourself what I am talking about. Remember the battle against your addictions is only fought in the beginning of your transition. Once you feel how good not eating that junk makes you feel, you will not be tempted again. Actually, it's better not to fight at all. Take the adversarial aspect of it out. Just reach for more of the good stuff and the desire for the bad stuff falls away on its own. The more of the good stuff you put in your body the less of the bad stuff you want. Many spiritual traditions have a tenant that goes something like "You do your 10% of the work necessary to transform spiritually, God's grace gives you the other 90%". This is the form that 90% takes. You lose the desire for the crap. It's not a constant battle of wills. Give your 10%, and the rewards will be beyond your wildest dreams.

If you can summon the will to begin the transition, you will be helped every step of the way. By whom? By you. The Masters tell us that we are enlightened already. There is nothing to get. There is nowhere to go. Only to realize you have it within yourself. They call it self-realization. Connecting with your own higher nature through the process of waking up your free will, of making your own choices, is a sure path to this realization. The path can be short or long, your choice. The way can be easy or hard. You decide.

I suggest you make it easy on yourself. Laugh at your failings. Smile at your triumphs. Jingle all the way. Relax into the process. Have fun awakening your inner power. Enjoy the dialogue between the part of you that feels stuck and addicted and the part that feels the pull to higher consciousness. Give more energy to the part of your psyche that wants to aspire to a new way of being. Put your focus on what you want. Never think you cannot have it. Enjoy the ride. Lighten up. Listen to your inner knowing. As Gandhi said, "Be the change you want to see in the world."

If being extremely healthy, extremely calm, extremely focused, and extremely vibrant makes me extreme in someone's eyes—so be it. I don't really care what others think of me. They're probably not watching anyway.

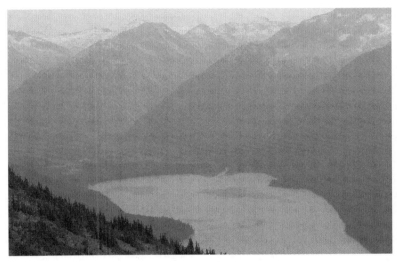

View of Cheakamus Lake from Whistler Mountain

"Creative minds have always been known to survive any kind of bad training."

- Anna Freud

CHAPTER 3
DEADLY DAIRY

M an is the only animal who consumes milk after weaning. We take the milk from another animal that weighs some 60 pounds at birth and weighs 600 in a few months. The milk of that animal is almost all fat, because fat is what is needed to build the big body. Human milk is almost all carbohydrate, because that's what is needed to build the big brain. Whose idea was this, to consume another animal's milk?

The fat in cow's milk is all omega 6, which is ubiquitous in the American diet and in all animal fat. The fat in human milk is 3, 9 and 7, very beneficial. In fact, these are all called essential fatty acids (EFAs).[1] They are essential fatty acids because your body doesn't make them and you must have them to live. Too much omega 6 in the diet increases inflammation and insulin resistance. This is the type of fat found in animal products. The average American gets way too much omega 6 and very little of the other omegas. The fat in dairy products, we do not need. It causes many problems in our bodies, not the least of which is occluded arteries. Butterfat,[2] the type found in dairy is more adept at clogging your arteries than any other type of fat except maybe trans (man-made) fat.[3]

Another problem with milk is the calcium, which is the wrong kind. Human bodies do not absorb it efficiently. Americans consume more dairy by far, than any other country per capita, yet we have the highest rate of osteoporosis.[4] A lot of new research is showing that unabsorbed calcium is a very bad thing, it forms the building material for all the stones like kidney, gall, and liver. There is a book entitled "The Liver and

Gallbladder Miracle Cleanse", by Andreas Moritz, that gives us a way to remove the stones from their hiding places.

New studies are showing that unabsorbed calcium also causes bone growth (ossification) in your arteries.[5] That's why "hardening of the arteries" happens. Bone material is forming in your arteries. The wrong kind of fat then sticks to this bone material forming a full or partial blockage in your arteries, which is the cause of stroke and most heart disease. You have been sold a very detrimental habit indeed.

New research is showing that this ossification is slowed down by adequate intake of vitamin K.[6] Vitamin K is in abundance in leafy greens. Other vegetables have it as well. If you going to continue to eat any amount of dairy, make sure you're getting lots of vitamin K. Some people eat only small amounts of dairy in salad dressing, cream in their coffee, etc. Be aware that any amount of this insidious nonfood will keep you on the fast track to decline. A little is better than a lot, but is very different from none. We have been taught that moderation is the key to health. Nothing could be further from the truth. Moderation is better than runaway indulgence, but a little of a substance as dangerous as dairy is still a one-way ticket to old age.

Dairy may well be the single biggest menace to health there is. People often tell me "I don't eat that much dairy". It doesn't take much dairy consumption to undermine your health in some very significant ways. I've been asked "which is worse, meat or dairy?" That's like asking "which is worse, heroin or cocaine?" Both will destroy your health in their own way. Like these drugs, a little is all it takes to cause major health problems and keep you on the fast track to aging.

Throughout this book when I talk about meat and the many dangers it poses to your health, I am also referring to dairy, fish, and eggs. They all attack your well-being the same way;

by filling your body with the wrong kind of fat, filling your arteries with cholesterol, polluting every cell in your body with toxins, and eroding away your quality of life. I am not overstating this. You will see when you get to the other side of your transition away from these horrible "nonfoods" just how good you can feel.

Keep in mind that eggs, though they may not carry quite the same toxic burden, as meat and dairy, are the richest source of cholesterol of any food.[7] You have no idea how wonderful you will feel when you cease putting all these unnatural foods into your body, and begin to cleanse out all the residue left behind by these insults to your health.

Dairy products and eggs are also the two "foods" that contribute the most to your bodily stores of "mucus", "phlegm", "catarrh". Whatever you want to call it, this stuff forms the perfect breeding ground for pathogens of all kinds. This is what comes out when you have a cold. It comes from all over the body, but when you blow it out your nose or spit it, that has come out of your lungs. We would drown in this sticky gooey substance if we did not get colds. Colds are actually cleanses. I haven't had one in many years, but if I did I would say I had a cleanse not a cold.[8] This is why they will never find a cure for the common cold. God forbid they ever do. You could drown on this stuff. When you stop the dairy and eggs and clean out the mucus they produced, you'll probably never have a cold again.

Speaking of colds, I have a great remedy for you. Not to "cure" the cleanse, but to enhance it, and shorten its duration. All you do to make it is blend fresh horseradish, garlic, ginger, white onion and jalapeno pepper. Put the mixture in a big glass bowl (or bowls) and add apple cider vinegar. Stir, cover the bowl, and leave overnight. Ladle off and strain the liquid. Add more apple cider vinegar and it will continue to absorb the ingredients. You can keep ladling off (or pouring through a strainer) and adding apple cider vinegar at least five or six times before it loses its punch. This is an excellent drink for detoxing purposes as well. You may find it hard to drink because it really packs a wallop. Mixing it with something like carrot juice works well. You have to sip it if you drink it straight, as if you're drinking strong whiskey. Cutting the ingredients into small pieces makes it a lot easier on your blender, even if you have a strong one like a Vita mix.

Remember there is nothing beneficial in any dairy product. There are a few nutrients in eggs but you can get those from many other sources without the huge hit of artery clogging cholesterol. You might think protein would be one benefit you could derive from a dairy product, but we already get too much.[9] Too much protein, as you will discover in a later chapter, is a very bad thing. Protein is something you get in abundance in any diet that includes enough calories to run the machine.

Some people cannot tolerate the sugar in dairy, called lactose. They are known as "lactose intolerant." Lucky them. Those who cannot consume dairy products have been spared a huge amount of wear and tear to the body. There are now "lactose free" dairy products available, and enzymes you can take to help deal with lactose. Rather than trying to make the body deal with dairy, these people should count their blessings.

Many people are allergic to dairy products. It is one of the most common allergens. Many others have a subclinical, in other words, not measurable allergic reaction to dairy products. What this means is an immune system compromised by these constant allergic irritations, but they don't realize it. Consumption of dairy products also increases allergies to other substances.

I worked with a lady a few years ago who was dreading the upcoming springtime allergy season. She was always severely affected, sneezing, and sniffling constantly in the springtime. I told her dairy consumption was probably the culprit. She told me she didn't eat much dairy, but then realized, oh yeah, cheese is dairy. She ate cheese virtually every day. I suggested that just as an experiment, that she stop eating cheese and all dairy to see what would happen. To say she was amazed by the result would be a supreme understatement. She called to tell me toward the end of allergy season that she sneezed maybe four times. She was extremely surprised and grateful. If you are affected by allergies– to anything, try quitting dairy.

Every time I have worked with someone who had allergies, and they were able to summon the will to quit dairy, the allergies disappeared. Even people who were plagued by multiple allergies found complete freedom from all allergic reaction by giving up dairy products. Bee pollen is very beneficial in helping with allergies, as it is gathered from flowers, and has a positive effect on the immune system. Nothing works to free you of allergies like giving up dairy. No substance be it natural or drug can enhance your immune system like completely giving up this insidious hazard to health.

I read of an experiment done on prisoners, wherein dairy products were removed from the prisoner's diets. The researchers noted the prisoners seemed much calmer. There were less fights and friction among the inmates after dairy was removed from their diets. We tend to think of dairy products as "comfort foods." I have clients tell me they felt much more peaceful when they removed this particular irritant. You can certainly add dairy products to the list of "comfort foods" that make us decidedly uncomfortable.

There is a huge advertising campaign on right now, touting chocolate milk as the perfect recovery food for athletes. They have triathletes, bicycle racers, and at least one speed skater, telling you this lie. It is claimed that chocolate milk has the perfect mix of carbohydrates, fat, and protein for recovery from intense exercise. Those of us have taken the time to learn a bit of nutritional science, know that butterfat, is very adept at clogging your circulatory system. The carbohydrates come from added sugar, which will cause glycation and many other health concerns. The protein? Let's just say there are a lot better ways to get yours. So much advertising now is aimed at people who have a more athletic lifestyle. I had to laugh at the latest Nature Valley granola bar commercial. It starts out with a couple standing by a waterfall and the voiceover saying, "It balances you" "it fills you with energy". OMG. I'm sure it's been shown in the laboratory to "balance you". Be careful. These messages get in there subliminally.

In his excellent book "Eat to Live," Dr. Fuhrman tells us "there is a strong association between dairy lactose and ischemic heart disease. There is also a clear association between high-growth promoting foods such as dairy products and cancer. There is a clear association between milk consumption and bladder, prostate, colorectal, and testicular cancers. Dairy fat is also loaded with various toxins and is the primary source of our nation's high exposure to dioxin. Dioxin is a highly toxic chemical compound that even the US environmental protection agency admits is a prominent cause of many types of cancer in those consuming dairy fat such as butter and cheese. Cheese is also a powerful inducer of acid load, which increases calcium loss further. Considering that cheese and butter are the foods with the highest saturated fat content and the major source of our dioxin exposure, cheese is particularly foolish choice for obtaining calcium".[10]

Dr. Fuhrman is showing us that milk, designed by nature to induce rapid growth, also hastens the growth of mutant cells—cancer. He also states that it boosts something called IGF-1, which stimulates the growth of both normal and cancer cells. He doesn't mention bovine growth hormone in this equation, but certainly, it plays a role in the growth of cancer cells also. So there you have it from an MD. Dairy = cancer. I like how he called eating cheese a "particularly foolish choice". I ask again, whose idea was this – to consume another animal's milk?

A great documentary to watch to further appreciate the damage meat and dairy do is "Forks over Knives". Another is "Sick Tired and Nearly Dead". Since the 70s I have seen the message that dairy is a destroyer of health go from fringe to almost mainstream. The dairy industry is working very hard to prevent this, but the truth is slowly leaking out. Also, check out the documentary "Food Inc."

I once saw a dollop of cheese from a pizza that was stuck to a plate. The plate was left under very hot water, directly under the stream of water. The water was blasting directly on the dollop of cheese. It was not budging. Just for fun, we left it like that for about 15 or 20 minutes. The cheese adhered to the plate no matter how much hot water was blasted onto it. I said to my friend "this is your arteries on cheese." It's hard to imagine anything more detrimental to your circulatory system than cheese, or more specifically, butterfat.

Another problem with consuming dairy is that it, like all animal "foods", creates an acid condition in the blood. It has long been known that the body will leach calcium from your bones to alkalinize your blood. The body must maintain a near neutral pH of around 7.[11] Now science is beginning to appreciate that in an overly acidic body, inflammation, stones of all types, arthritis, high blood pressure, chronic fatigue and irritability as well as calcium leaching is bound to occur. It has even been said that no disease can exist in an alkaline environment.

Soft drinks, with a pH of 2, and high levels of phosphoric acid, especially in dark colas, represent a serious threat to your bones and overall state of health. Other highly acidic drinks are beer with a pH of 2.5, and our beloved coffee, with a pH of 4. Alcoholic beverages of all kinds are acidifying. Interesting to note, a pH of 6 is 6 to 10 times more acidic than a pH of 7.[12] Does this mean that you can't have your coffee? No. If you're eating foods that are predominantly alkalinizing, then you don't have to worry so much about consuming acidifying drinks.

Fermented foods of all kinds are alkalinizing.[13] Fruits and vegetables, which hopefully you will be consuming a lot of after you give up animal foods are alkalinizing as well as nourishing. Nuts and seeds also score well into the alkaline zone. Beans not so much, but again, if you're consuming predominantly alkalinizing food, you don't need to worry. Having a "balanced pH", or in other words a neutral pH, has been shown to stimulate fat burning. Definitely a good thing. What we are doing as age reversers, is weeding out the foods that were aging us, and eating as much as we want of the foods that will strengthen us. Easy.

A substance in Basil called eugenol[14] has been shown to slow the inflammation caused by dairy and other animal foods. It may also stimulate blood sugar stabilization. This is a wonderful herb to cook with and to take in supplement form. We must do everything we can to undo the damage caused by consumption of animal products.

Years ago, I read that cow's milk contains a substance called lactomorphine[15] Recently I heard it referred to as Quesomorphine. Cows were originally prey animals, and in many prey species, the survival strategy for newborns is to lay still to avoid being spotted by predators. It could be that this substance has evolved to keep the baby calm. In humans, this substance helps account for the addictive nature of dairy products.

When you wean yourself off this insidious nonfood, you will be on your way to recapturing your youth. You may well go beyond the feeling of youthfulness you had when you were young. You may find you feel better than you ever felt in your life—even in your youth. This nonfood was aging you at an accelerated rate. When you get dairy products completely out of your diet, the party can really start... without the morphine.

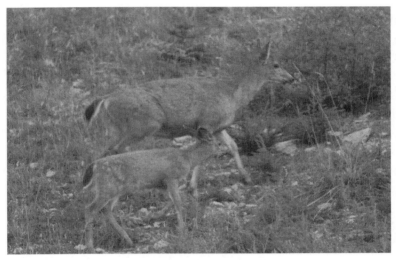

Blacktail deer of Whistler

"If you limit your choices to only what seems possible or reasonable, you disconnect yourself from what you truly want and all that is left is a compromise."

- Elaine Borish

CHAPTER 4
MEAT: DEATH IN, DEATH OUT

We are not carnivores. Of course, you know that. What you may not know is that we're not omnivores either. Omnivores, like bears and raccoons, have a carnivore's digestive system. Their adaptation to eating plant material is grinding teeth in the rear of their jaws. What's a carnivore's digestive system you ask? It is characterized by a short small intestine and no colon. Instead the large intestine is a belling-out of the small intestine. It is smooth, with no convolutions as our large intestine (colon) has. It's not expandable as ours is. That's why when your dog has to go, he can't hold it for long like you can.

There seem to be 4 basic designs in mammal digestive systems. The herbivore, with its 4 stomachs, the carnivore/omnivore, the frugivore, like the great apes, and us. We are unique. Even though chimps famously share 90% of our DNA, we have something they don't have. The colon. A wonderful adaptation, but things can go wrong—seriously wrong with it.[1]

This organ gives the human animal the most endurance in the heat of any animal in the world as long as we have sufficient water. Also, being naked helps (no hair on our bodies), because we're able to dissipate heat through sweating, using the whole body as a thermoregulator. The colon acts as a canteen, storing and absorbing water. In fact, all of the liquid you drink is absorbed through the walls of the colon. Trouble is, the colon is also the last stop in the digestive system. What's wrong with this picture? The organ that absorbs all your liquid is the organ where the "do-do" is hanging out, and it ain't getting any fresher.[2]

In fact, if your colon is like most peoples, you might as well be drinking out of the toilet. This explains why colon cancer is now the #3 killer in this country. It explains why cancer of all kinds are so prevalent. We are constantly reabsorbing toxins our bodies are trying to get rid of. Some carcinogens come from the environment undoubtedly, but many types of cancer originate in the poor neglected colon. It is a breeding ground for pathogens and mutant cells. So little is appreciated about this process, but it doesn't take the proverbial rocket scientist to see that the colon must be cleansed for us to be able not to worry about cancer. The idea that the colon is filthy is actually good news! It means that if you cleanse the colon, you won't have to worry about these "mysterious" diseases. It means that if you clean it up, you won't age at the normal fast rate.[3]

Another adaptation that proves we are not omnivores is the fact that carnivores/omnivores manufacture Vitamin C in their own bodies. We, on the other hand will die without it. Since our natural foods are rich in Vitamin C, there was no need for our bodies to evolve to make it. Nature is very efficient like that.[4]

Omnivores share the same sharp teeth with the carnivores. They all have canines—fangs. The difference is that omnivores have grinders too. Many of them eat mostly vegetable matter. We have no sharp teeth or claws. We can't process meat well without it being cooked. We actually don't process it well, period.

Further proof that we are not omnivores is our low protein requirement. In us, too much protein is a very dangerous thing—on many levels. First is the fact that too much protein causes an acid condition in the blood. The body cannot tolerate this, and will do whatever it takes to raise the pH in whatever way it can, as fast as it can—regardless of the cost to the body. It has to—you'll die if it doesn't.

The quickest way to raise your blood pH, it turns outs, is to leach calcium from your bones. This helps explain the epidemic of osteoporosis, in this and other "developed" countries. The simple fact is that dead, decaying flesh cannot do anything but destroy your health.[5]

New research is showing that it's worse than we thought. When meat is cooked at high temperatures, the protein is denatured. Worse still is a newly appreciated substance called arachnadonic acid. Arachnadonic acid gets its name from its resemblance to a spider's web as it forms structures in the tissues. It has been shown to increase inflammation and has been linked to many disease systems, high blood pressure, thrombosis (blood clots), allergic reaction, arthritis, depression, and other widely varied health concerns. Another serious health hazard that you eat directly from meat is AGEs— advanced glycation end products. I have a whole chapter about AGEs coming up for you.[6]

Animals and humans have evolved no mechanism to deal with the unbelievable spectrum of industrial pollutants in our world now. These toxins have only been in the environment for a generation or so. There are new ones every day, especially antibiotics, which have to be changed—made stronger to keep pace with the rapid evolution of pathogens. These organisms adapt to the latest antibiotic very quickly, so stronger ones are always needed in order to raise animals in close confinement. Pesticides are also necessary in huge amounts in any feedlot or chicken house. We've all heard of growth hormones, particularly BGH, (bovine growth hormone). Can't lose weight? Uh yeah, you're eating massive amounts of growth hormone.[7]

Since we animals have evolved no mechanism for getting rid of toxins, we don't. We store them throughout the body particularly in our fat. When you eat a piece of meat, even grass fed or "free range", you are getting all the toxins that animal ever ate; it ate a lot. The animal on the top of the food chain gets all the toxins that all the animals that it ever ate consumed throughout their lives. So if you get the picture that a beef cow or chicken is a veritable storehouse of all kinds of poisons, and that when you eat those poisons you become unbelievably toxic, imagine if something were eating us. That animal would probably have a very short life. If a grizzly bear or a shark were to eat enough human flesh, it would probably just drop over dead. We need to get to the bottom of the food chain as quickly as possible.[8]

The fact that animal bodies have not evolved a system to get rid of toxins is highly significant. It means that animals store the toxins in their tissues that they have been exposed to. It means also when we eat these animals we not only inherit their stored toxins, but that we will not get rid of them either. The lymphatic system, the body's "other" circulatory system, is our main waste disposal pathway. Today's toxins easily overwhelm it. Lymphoma or lymphatic cancer is one symptom of an overwhelmed lymphatic system.

I will have much more to say throughout this book on the many hazards meat consumption poses to our health. Of the many ways the body is attacked, be it by occlusion of our arteries, high cholesterol, advanced glycation end products, acid condition in the blood, this list could go on and on; the bloody hands of meat consumption are on you! You will never know how good your body can feel until you get the residue from meat out of your body. All of the aforementioned hazards to your health, and many more besides, are the residue of meat consumption.

Become part of the solution. Stop the cruelty and exploitation of animals. It is unbelievable how we treat them. We're shown Humane Society commercials of animals neglected and abused, but nothing is said about the much more numerous "farm" animals that are hideously slaughtered every minute of every day, and kept in unbelievably cruel conditions.

The poor dairy cows have it much worse. Instead of being killed at several months of age, they have to endure their torturous existence for years, not to mention being genetically and chemically manipulated to give upwards of a hundred gallons of milk a day.[9]

The law of cause and effect says something like "you reap what you sew." Every religion has a variation on this. All the suffering we subject these animals to is returned to us. We kill and subjugate them, and they kill us slowly when we're selfish and foolish enough to eat them. Not to mention the environmental cost.

It's been said that one cow emits more greenhouse gas in a year than an SUV (through farts). That's because methane, the gas that they emit is many times worse than CO_2. That says nothing of the vast mounds of manure from feedlots that are also outgassing methane into the air.

Chicken and hog "farms" are even worse. Many rural families have had their well water rendered undrinkable by runoff from hog and chicken operations. By the way, do you know what "free range" means? I've heard that to qualify under USDA's definition, it's a chicken that has been raised in a chicken house with a window. Try quitting meat and feel the difference. Become part of your own solution as well as the solution to the huge environmental issues we face.[10]

One reason meat has been embraced as a healthy food is because for years it was thought that in order to absorb the protein in a food; all eight of the essential amino acids that your body cannot manufacture needed to be present. This was known as a "complete protein.[11]" It was thought that if you ate food that had an incomplete protein profile, you would not be able to benefit from the protein in that food. All animal foods offer a complete protein profile, and therefore were thought to be superior sources of protein.

Soy is one non-animal food (besides spirolina and chia seeds) that contains a complete protein, and is one reason that it is touted as a health food. One of the early books on vegetarianism called "Diet for a Small Planet," which was one of the earliest treatises on the environmental destruction meat production causes, also perpetuated this myth. There was a follow-up book called "Recipes for a Small Planet," which offered recipes that would "balance" the amino acids consumed at a meal, so that a complete protein could be made out of two foods that had incomplete protein profiles. An example could be corn and beans. One has certain amino acids, the other "complements" or completes the other's amino acid profiles to achieve a complete protein. This is a myth that is not completely dead. Some still talk about which foods go with which, to achieve a complete protein.

The whole concept has been shown to be absolute rubbish. If this were true half the human population in the world would be protein deficient. There are so many myths that are perpetuated. Many populations throughout the world for example, eat no protein other than that contained in rice.

Of course I have to jump on this, and say that if a complete protein were necessary for human nutrition, it might prove that we do well on a meat diet. The fact that this is balderdash points to the fact that we are not omnivores.

There have been some books recently that advocate a return to our hunter-gatherer diets - no wheat or dairy. Just remember, any diet that advocates eating meat because our ancestors did is missing something. What? The fact that meat and fish as well as eggs and dairy are full of toxins. They are not our natural food. Yes, man has been eating meat for thousands of years, but that doesn't mean it's something we should keep doing. We've also been killing each other and are now threatening life on Earth. We've done a lot of dumb stuff. Meat, in our hunter-gatherer days was the only food that was available at least some of the year. We can now choose the foods that will really sustain us.

When you eat animal foods, toxins build up in your fat, liver, and indeed every cell in your body. An animal who consumes antibiotics and growth hormone carries vast stores of them in their tissues. When you eat their dead bodies, you get a massive hit of antibiotics that you are now the proud owner of. The body does not secrete these readily. These antibiotics, growth hormones, pesticides, etc. are not something the body ever evolved to deal with. No mechanism exists in the body for ridding it of these toxins.[12]

Likewise, the fish those of us who are not informed eat are full of toxins. There are no clean fish left in any ocean. Fish samples from Antarctica, as far away from civilization as you can get, show high concentrations of the entire spectrum of industrial pollutants. The oceans are never static. There are currents (like the Gulf Stream) at all depths of the ocean. The water that is in the Boston Harbor today, two years later is in Antarctica. Pollutants such as mercury, lead, cadmium, and arsenic have been shown to be highly toxic to all body tissues, especially the brain. These build up in our brains just as they do in the fish. The bigger the fish the more toxins it contains. The older the animal the more time it has had to store these toxins and the more revenge it takes on us for killing and eating its dead body.[13]

In this regard, chicken is better for you than beef. It's killed at six weeks instead of several months of age. Therefore, chicken has had less time to accumulate toxins like antibiotics and pesticides.

Fish accumulate toxins from the water they live in very efficiently because they are always surrounded by this water. They are taking up toxins not only by eating them, but by breathing them as well. Just about all fish eat other fish. There are a few species like parrotfish that graze on algae. Most eat other fish every day of their lives. In so doing they eat the concentrations of toxins that those fish contain. The older the fish, the more toxins it has ingested and concentrated. If you must eat fish, eat small ones like sardines and anchovies. The big predatory fish like tuna, swordfish, or mackerel carry the biggest toxic burden.

From an artery, clogging standpoint fish is certainly better than beef or chicken. The fat in fish is actually beneficial, which is the reason so many people take fish oil as a dietary supplement.

You can handle fish, and then rinse your hands off; your hands may have a little fishy smell but they will not feel greasy. Try that after handling meat or cheese. You will never get that waxy grease off your hands without soap and hot water. This is showing what the fat in meat and dairy does in your arteries.

If we had to kill and clean all that fish and meat we ate, there would be a whole lot more vegetarians. Would you be able to chop a chicken's head off and then get its blood all over your hands? Didn't think so. When we contribute to their suffering, we suffer. When you stop contributing to their horrible treatment, you feel a new kinship with all of creation.

I know, here I go again, but what about you? Are you a Christian? One of the Ten Commandments is thou shalt not kill. It doesn't say thou shalt not kill people, but that killing is wrong. One of the first lines in the bible in the book of Genesis says "Behold I give you every herb bearing seed and, to you, it shall be for meat." All deeper spiritual paths have non killing (ahimsa) at their center. Why? Because eating death makes you fretful and afraid. Remember, these animals are killed on an assembly line. Their meat is full of adrenaline. Eat their fear. You'll be afraid. If you're afraid, you can be controlled. The meat is also a repository for every antibiotic, growth hormone and pesticide the animal has ever ingested.

What about grass fed beef and free-range chicken? It's gotta be better, right? Maybe, but it will still contain toxins. It will still create an acid condition in the blood, which will result in calcium leaching. It will still clog your arteries. It will still not allow you to age in reverse. You can slow down the aging process by eating so-called organic meat, dairy and eggs and taking supplements. Eat less crap and of course, aging is slowed down comparatively. I'm not writing a book about slowing down the aging process but one about reversing it. There is a huge difference. Aging in reverse is not possible if you continue to go against your nature. We are not omnivores.

A major ingredient of commercial animal feed is "byproducts"- ground-up bone, skin, hooves, etc. Cattle raised in feedlots, as 99% of them are, are cannibals. They are fed a "slurry", a liquid feed consisting of corn and grain, but also blood, and other disgusting leftovers from processing. It's been said that 1% of the beef grown in America ever sees a blade of grass. Cattle are raised in huge feedlots, where hundreds of animals are kept in a series of corrals laid out in a grid pattern. It takes massive amounts of antibiotics to keep animals in these close quarters. A modern chicken house can have upwards of 10,000 chickens housed in it. Like a feedlot, if one got sick, they would all get sick. These animals are fed unbelievable amounts of antibiotics, which are absolutely proven to be stored in the animal's body. When you eat these animals, you get huge concentrations of antibiotics.

You may have heard the term "super germ."[14] This term refers to bacteria that have evolved resistance to antibiotics. These organisms have a very short life, and are able to pass on mutations to future generations very quickly. This is how they have evolved for millions of years. We are speeding up their evolution by introducing challenges to these bacteria in the form of antibiotics. They are very well able to rise to the occasion. As we try to eradicate these bacteria with antibiotics, they respond by becoming stronger and more vigorous. This could prove to be a huge problem one day, if things continue as they are. To keep pace with these mutations–these adaptations the bacteria are able to go through; science has to keep changing up the antibiotics. Science mostly changes them one way–by making them stronger and stronger. Our children are the first generation ever to be raised on massive amounts of antibiotics. What this will do to them, we have no idea. We are all guinea pigs...well most of us.

The Food and Drug Administration, Federal Trade Commission and U.S. Department of Agriculture are not in the business of safeguarding your health. They are in the business of protecting the profits of drug companies and food producers while raking in huge profits for number one. And, number one ain't you...you ain't even number two.

Witness the attack on our health freedom by trying to outlaw, directly or indirectly, all herbs, and supplements. It almost happened in 1994. A move was narrowly defeated to outlaw herbs and supplements except as prescribed by a doctor. There is a move afoot now to severely curtail our health freedom in the same way. Thomas Jefferson said, "The price of freedom is eternal vigilance."

The latest attack is CODEX, a thinly disguised attempt to eliminate the competition for the drug companies and to strip you of remedies that work. It is law in parts of Europe where it has raised the price of supplements quite a bit. Certain Senators led by Dick Durbin are seeking to "harmonize" with the CODEX laws of Europe. Google CODEX and see what I mean.[15]

Mad Cow disease is mentioned now and then in the news, popping up somewhere else followed by the assurance that the U.S. doesn't have it. Most people don't know what Mad Cow disease is. If you ask them they would probably say it's a virus or something - it's not. Mad Cow disease is caused by protein called a mutant prion. Virtually indestructible, they represent an entirely different class of pathogen. Not a living organism, the abnormal version of a protein known as a prion is able to withstand conditions, which kill any other pathogen. They have the ability to withstand temperatures of over 1100°F, evade the immune system, and replicate themselves. Bacteria and viruses are killed by high temperatures. This mis-folded molecule that destroys brain tissue is not alive, and so cannot be killed. Abnormal prions mutate neighboring prions upon contact, causing them to fold improperly and mutate their neighbors in a domino effect.

Unlike normal prions, mutants do not break down when meat is digested. The immune system is not provoked to attack the invader, because normal and rogue prions are almost chemically identical. When humans get this disease, it is called Creutzfeldt-Jakob disease. The incubation period can be 30 years or more. I wanted to tell you a little bit about what this disease is and that you can't rely on those who are in the business of protecting industry to protect you. Here again, education is the key. Knowledge is power. Ignorance is anything but bliss. Alzheimer's looks in an MRI a lot like

Creutzfeldt-Jakob disease. It may be that some of what is being called Alzheimer's is really C. J. disease.[16]

No worries, anything can be regenerated, as long as enough life force exists in the body. People have cured so many supposedly incurable diseases; the term incurable is almost meaningless. If we stop putting things in our bodies that age us and cause disease, our diseases will begin to heal of their own accord. Remove the caustic irritants from your vehicle and it will be a whole lot more fun to drive. So many people worry about things they can do nothing about. So many people do nothing about things they should worry about. Actually, worry is useless. What we need is action. Discernment. A bit of willpower. Or maybe won't power.

We are creatures of habit. We are naturally creatures with complete and utter free will. You can recapture and revitalize your free will by using it, by seeing how you have been manipulated, how you have been conditioned, and how you have been complacent. By establishing new habits. The rewards are so great for waking up. A book like this is of no value, unless it can inspire you to make these changes.

Yes, knowledge is power and education is the key. You have the power to unlock your potential. Free will is the hand that turns the key. The lock, as you will find out, is of your own making. You did have some help in making this lock, but now, if you use the key, you will be free. Free to choose. Free to be an inspiration to everyone in your sphere of influence, which means everyone, everywhere.

Quantum physics shows us that we are not in a machine that has been switched on and left to run. We are part of a giant organism, and that one part of this organism influences the whole thing. We influence each other; we influence the mass consciousness, to a degree you probably have not appreciated. As you feel better and better physically, your capacity to care grows exponentially. If you are not a kind, compassionate spirit, you will be, and not a moment too soon. If we are to survive as a species, we must become much nicer; Nicer to the planet, nicer to our fellow creatures and especially nicer to ourselves.

As you clean up your diet, and your vehicle starts running a whole lot better, you will be inspired as never before to be part of the solution. By choosing cleaner food, you choose a cleaner world. For instance, much of the Western United States, including many major cities, relies on the Colorado River. So much so that the Colorado runs out of water over 100 miles before it reaches the sea. 70% of the Colorado River water is used for growing crops for animal feed. One hamburger requires 500 gallons of this precious resource to produce. If each person in America ate one fewer hamburger a year, we could restore flow to the lower Colorado.[17]

Water is soon to be in short supply. Aquifers (underground reservoirs) are being sucked dry at a phenomenal rate. Glaciers are melting which supply water to well over a third of the world's population. We may soon be in shallow water and deep doo-doo. If you live in a coastal city, you may be in deep salt water. We have a lot of work to do, if we want to leave a habitable world to our children and our future selves.

There is no better place to start than in your own environment (your body). It sounds like a lot of work to wake up, to become more aware, to become more compassionate, and to care more. It's not. It's who you are. Get rid of the caustic irritants you consume on a daily basis. You will be amazed at how simple it is to do, and how powerful these substances are. But, you are more powerful; hopefully, you are becoming empowered to clean this crap out of your life once and for all. Make a firm resolution. If you break it, don't worry. Just start again.

In Alcoholics Anonymous, they don't tell you to cut down on alcohol. They tell you to stop. Speaking of alcohol, I'm not suggesting you have to give up all alcohol, but you probably will eventually. When you have a good buzz going on, you won't want anything that takes you out of it. When your body is clean and you drink alcohol you will feel it—and not in a good way.

In AA, when you fall off the wagon, you start all over again. You're only clean and sober since your last drink. I don't go with that. Falling off the wagon and getting back on is all part of it. If you stop eating meat, for instance, then in a moment of weakness or to appease someone else, you eat some, this will strengthen your resolve not to eat meat again because it will make you feel tired and lethargic for days or weeks after you eat it. The longer you go not eating meat, the more you'll feel it when you do. You will be inspired not to eat dead decaying flesh again.

When I was eighteen, I saw meat as disgusting, once I realized how bad it was for me. I was never tempted to eat it again. Dairy was a different story. I did have a problem kicking ice cream. It was my weakness. The longer I went between binges, the worse ice cream made me feel when I ate it, especially the next day. Finally, one day, I had my last binge. You never know when the last one will be. Be gentle with yourself. Balance that with pushing yourself to be better and better. When you feed the addiction, you will have the addiction.

There's no need to wean yourself slowly off this stuff, but remember, the bad food is so toxic, that by stopping, you will go into detox mode. Don't let this derail you. Many have fallen into the trap of feeling bad when they stop eating the junk, and concluding that they need meat or whatever to feel good. This is an honest mistake. You may find you feel great when you first quit the junk, but then, usually around the three-week mark, you may feel tired or irritable. This feeling is because you have given your body some breathing room, you stopped putting the heavy toxic crap into it, and it is endeavoring to clean up the mess. Again, the body has not really evolved to do this, but does the best it can. If you feel bad, your body is showing how toxic your body has gotten. Eating the junk again will stop that process, and you may feel better. Don't fall into this trap.

Instead, drink lots of juice, as that will hydrate you and help you flush the toxins. It will also give you the antioxidants and carbs to keep going. Yes, some juices do have too many carbs to be a regular part of your diet, but right now, you need all the help you can get. Sometimes, carbohydrates are not such a bad thing. Be sure to let yourself rest when you need to. Above all, don't forget the enemas and maybe treat yourself to a colonic or 10, but more about these later. Don't worry; this is going to be fun. No, not the enema, the feeling better part. The enemas are just part of what it takes to get you there easily and gently.

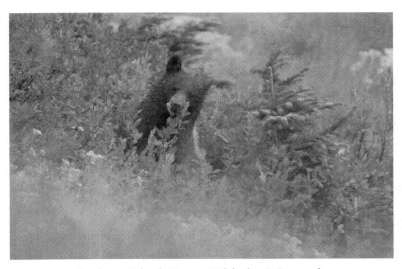

Curious Black Bear, Whistler Mountain

"Unexplored paths lead to undiscovered treasures."

\- Constance Chuks Friday

CHAPTER 5
PROTEIN—HOW MUCH IS TOO MUCH?

A quote from our friend Dr. Joel Furhman: "Scientific studies provide evidence that animal protein's effect on blood cholesterol may be significant. This is one of the reasons that those switching to a low-fat diet do not experience the cholesterol lowering they expect unless they also remove low-fat animal products as well. Surprising to most people is that yes even low-fat dairy and skinless white meat chicken raise cholesterol. I see this regularly in my practice. Many individuals do not see the dramatic drop in cholesterol levels unless they go all the way and remove all animal protein from their diet." He also states, "Chicken has the same amount of cholesterol as beef and that the production of these potent cancer-causing compounds called heterocyclic amines (HCAs) are even more concentrated in grilled chicken then in beef. Another study from New Zealand that investigated HCAs in meat, fish, and chicken found the greatest contributor of HCAs to cancer risk was chicken. Likewise, studies indicate that chicken is almost as dangerous as red meat for the heart. Regarding cholesterol, there is no advantage to eating lean white instead of lean red meat. The best bet for overall health is to significantly limit or eliminate all types of meat—red and white."

The above-mentioned quote was made by an MD who is not given to sweeping generalizations. As you can tell from his wording, he is very careful not to sound "absolute" or overly emphatic. We see in his words evidence that not only does meat cause heart disease but cancer as well. I am going to go into the meat-cancer connection in more depth later. I include this quote primarily to hip you to the fact that chicken, which is enjoying a surge of popularity these days due to its supposed health benefits over beef, is actually as bad or worse. Indeed, there is no animal "food" that can do anything but destroy your health and accelerate all aging processes. Remember what he said about fish. "You could drink water from the Great Lakes for 100 years and not get the same concentration of toxins you would get from eating 1 pound of fish from these lakes."

How much protein do we actually need, and how are we to get it if we don't consume animal products? Turns out just about all foods have protein. If we stop consuming animal products, we will not be getting the massive concentrations of protein that most Americans consume. This will prove to increase our quality of life significantly. The new consensus among more enlightened doctors and health educators is that— drumroll please—if you are eating a diet that supplies enough calories to meet your metabolic need for energy, you are getting enough protein. Bottom line. End of story. We must be concerned very much about protein. We must not get too much.

We have been conditioned to think we need massive amounts of protein to be healthy. We have been brainwashed to believe that we must have a "complete protein", and that animal products are the only place to get this. That much is true, animal products are virtually the only source of complete protein. As any health educator who is not in the Stone Age will tell you; to the body there is no such thing as a complete protein. All protein is broken down into its constituent parts— individual amino acids. So a complete protein is not only unnecessary, but from a metabolic standpoint, it is not even possible.[1]

I read in the 1970s about how a coach for the Pittsburgh Steelers decided to experiment on his players by drastically reducing their protein intake. He noticed almost immediately the players had more endurance and energy, and their injury rate went way down. Virtually any athlete who experiments with lowering his protein intake has noticed a huge improvement in endurance and energy level. For athletes the bottom line is the same as for regular people: if you have an adequate diet, you have an adequate protein intake. Athletes may need to eat more than regular folks do. If they do, they will automatically be getting more protein.

No need to assign a number of grams of protein we need each day. The new research is showing us we need not worry about our protein intake as long as we are eating sufficient calories to get us through the day. This is not new knowledge. It is however, only seeing the light of day on a large scale recently.

John Robbins in his book "Diet for a New America" shows us some examples of how the meat, dairy, and egg industries have continually suppressed information and perverted facts to support their claim that these nonfoods are essential to health, and that their products are safe. You may recall how in the 90s Oprah was sued by the beef industry for merely suggesting that Americans eat less beef. She won the suit but it cost her millions in legal fees.[2] Many other people without such deep pockets have been permanently silenced. Threatening someone as they have many times, with legal action is usually enough to stop them talking about the dangers these nonfoods pose.

Some people like to assign a number value to the amount of nutrients we should be getting. When it comes to protein this number would be how many grams of protein we need. Since we don't need to be concerned with getting enough, let's put a gram value on how much is too much. Actually, the body has done that for us. Since the 80s, science has known that the maximum amount of protein the average body can process at any one time is 30 grams. This is equal to the amount contained in a small can—one of those little lunch cans, of tuna.[3]

This finding influenced many athletes in the 80s, particularly bodybuilders. It changed the game completely. No more are bodybuilders eating huge amounts of protein at a time, as they did in the 60s and 70s. It has become the new conventional wisdom in bodybuilding to eat 6 to 8 small meals a day, some of which are protein shakes.

There is still some controversy about how much protein the body can process at a time. There may be some folks who can process more due to training or genetics. The consensus that I've observed through my research is that 30 grams is pretty much it. To my individual body 30 grams would be an absurdly huge amount. I get a fraction of that in a day and am putting on muscle at a very gratifying rate. People ask me how I can put on so much muscle on so little protein. Uh…it's called working out.

Athletes are always looking for an edge. I was just reading about how extreme endurance athletes, like the folks who run ultra-marathons and races like the Western States 100, are experimenting with high fat intake as a fuel source. The more enlightened ones will no doubt be looking to healthy fats like nuts and seeds, avocado, and healthy oils. Endurance athletes can eat lots of unhealthy fat without getting fat themselves, due to their high requirement for calories to fuel their long workouts. It turns out that fat packs a lot more calories than carbohydrates. This is good news for endurance athletes, but if they get their fat from animal sources, they will be clogging their arteries and eroding their quality of life just as surely as regular folks.

It's not protein that builds body tissues; it is specific amino acids among other things. These are: creatine, glutamine, carnitine, carnosine, and the three "branched chain" aminos, leucine, isoleucine and valine.[4]

I am asked all the time where I get protein since I've been on a liquid diet for 17 years. Heck, I used to get asked that question when I was just vegetarian. So strong is this belief that we need massive amounts. Why is this belief so widespread? The foods with the highest profit margins to the purveyors are meat and dairy. Did you know that the USDA buys up all the surplus milk produced in this country to keep the price artificially high?[5] Yep, sad but true. It is turned into cheese and used in school lunch programs and other subsidized government programs and stored in vast refrigerated warehouses at taxpayer's expense.

These industries are very powerful. You could say they ARE the government, but that's another story. Suffice to say we are not given the real facts in many instances. Roswell and 911? Never mind. Let's just say we have to educate ourselves. That's why you're reading this book. Trust yourself to find what's real in this sea of information we're floating in.

So, how much protein do we need? Not that much. Current research seems to be bringing the amount down fast. For instance, starvation used to be called kwashiorkor, which means protein deficiency. Now it's known as marasmus. Which means, "body wasting." This is now known to be caused by carbohydrate deficiency. The body thrives best on clean burning energy. This is not today's high protein foods by any stretch of the imagination.

Another amino worth mentioning is taurine. Known as the antioxidant amino, it protects the body from environmental toxins; both self-inflicted and otherwise. You may want to supplement these amino acids in your quest to build muscle. My favorite recovery supplement is NAC, n-acetyl cysteine. Cysteine is one of the eight essential amino acids that our bodies don't manufacture. There are 22 (some say 20) amino acids that comprise protein. We can produce all but eight ourselves. Anyway, NAC is an amazing substance. One of the things it does for us is to supply the liver with the raw material to produce glutathione, which is your body's master antioxidant. More on NAC later.

Here's a quote from "Diet for a New America": "The calcium lost from your bones due to excess protein has to go somewhere after it has served its purpose in our bloodstreams (lowering PH due to too much protein). So does the calcium we have ingested but have not been able to absorb due to high phosphorus/calcium ratios (like cow's milk). It all ends up in our urine, producing very high levels of calcium in the kidney system and all too often crystallizing into kidney stones. This is why kidney stones, the most painful of all medical emergencies, are seen far more frequently in meat eaters than in vegetarians. People who have suffered kidney damage or loss are usually able to preserve their remaining kidney function only if they are put on a protein-restricted diet. Those kidney patients whose protein intake is not restricted, particularly those who continue to eat meat, show rapid deterioration of their kidneys to the point where they may become dependent on kidney dialysis machines."

A further quote from that book: "The digestion of meat produces strong carcinogenic substances in the colon and meat eaters must produce excessive bile acids in their intestines to deal with the meat they eat, particularly deoxycholic acid. This is extremely significant because deoxycholic acid is converted by clostridia bacteria into powerful carcinogens in our intestines. The fact that meat eaters invariably have far more deoxycholic acid in their intestines than do vegetarians is one of the reasons they have so much higher rates of colon cancer."

The knowledge that too much protein causes a host of health conditions is becoming almost mainstream these days. In the Journal of the American Medical Association, an article appeared talking about how high animal protein diets measurably shorten the life spans of a number of different animals. It stated, "These findings corroborate the world health statistics that show human meat eating populations do not, as a rule, live as long as vegetarian populations."

Let me state one more time, just to make sure we're clear, too much protein in the diet causes an acid condition in the blood. The body cannot tolerate an acid condition in the blood, and so leaches calcium from the bones to alkalinize the blood, to attain a near neutral pH of around seven. In other words, the body steals calcium from your bones when you get too much protein in your diet. Osteoporosis is all but guaranteed.

We now understand that too much protein equals bone loss, many types of cancer, and cardiovascular complications in many forms. You don't have to look too far for this information nowadays. If you do your own experimentation, you will find, as these researchers have found—everything works better when you don't overload your body with protein. Give yourself the gift of virtually limitless energy and age reversal. It may take time to clear out the residue and byproducts accrued by a higher protein diet. Just by eating a lot less, they will begin to clear themselves from your machine. It will then run a lot better for a lot longer.

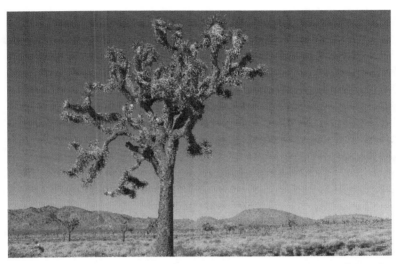

Joshua Tree in Joshua Tree National Monument, California

"Life isn't about finding yourself. Life is about creating yourself."

- George Bernard Shaw

CHAPTER 6
WHEAT IS NO TREAT

Now on to your wheat addiction. If you don't have one, don't take offense. Chances are you do, and it's aging you at an incredibly accelerated rate. I quit wheat as a young dude when I read about how the gluten in it is like glue in your colon and how fattening it is. Lucky me. Now we're discovering many, many more reasons to put this stuff where it belongs—in the garbage.

Wheat gluten triggers inflammation. One piece of bread impedes zinc and iron absorption by 90%. Gluten also contains an opiate which causes withdrawal symptoms.

Turns out, wheat is the single most fattening thing you can consume. I'm not talking white bread either. Whole wheat is just as bad at spiking your blood sugar. These blood sugar spikes do harm in ways we're only now starting to appreciate. First, your body has to put out this inflammatory fire. It does that through insulin, which the pancreas makes and secretes. Just as your body has no real capacity to process dead, decaying flesh, it has no defense against this insult either.[1] We simply didn't need to evolve a defense against these assaults because they don't exist in nature. Nothing in nature causes these dangerous spikes. Yes, whole wheat bread doesn't occur in nature. It's man made. The sugar in it is worse than pure table sugar.

Table sugar (sucrose) is a disaccharide or two sugar molecules – fructose and glucose. So it's absorbed through both the liver and the gut. The sugar in bread, pasta, and all of those hideous flour products is a monosaccride– glucose. This goes straight into the blood stream and causes an inflammatory fire in the form of a surge in blood sugar. The pancreas dumps a bunch of insulin in to quell these blood sugar spikes. Insulin, interestingly enough, also causes the body to store fat. Again, the body has no adaptation to this form of abuse. Here is an example of another lack of adaptation–you have no capacity to release this excess sugar. The body evolved to be very efficient–to survive in times of scarcity. No human in all of human evolution ever ate every day, or kept fat on the body all year round, except in recent times.[2]

We've evolved many strategies to keep fat on our bodies until needed. Insulin has many properties. One is to help the body conserve precious resources. What happens eventually, due to these daily blood sugar spikes is that like a drug, your body forms a tolerance to insulin, and so needs more of it to have an effect. The insulin receptors actually start to shut down, you stop responding to it, so the pancreas pumps out more. This is the beginning of the newly termed "metabolic syndrome"—and syndrome it is. When you have it, your body has become a fat storing machine. It will even take circulating ATP—your fuel—and put it in your fat cells. This is why a hallmark of metabolic syndrome is low energy. You might think your overweight friend is just tired from carrying all that extra weight around. No, he has become a fat storing machine.[3] Circulating ATP is being shuttled into his fat cells whether he needs it for energy or not. This leaves him severely depleted of energy.

Just about all of us abuse carbohydrates, and just about all of us have metabolic syndrome to some degree. It's also known as pre-diabetes. Full blown diabetes is also known as "adult onset" diabetes. Now it's not so much adult onset as it used to be. Now many kids have it too. As you will learn from the documentary "Food Inc.", 1 in 3 kids born since 2000 will develop diabetes. When you have diabetes, you have to inject insulin, because now you need massive amounts—so much your poor abused pancreas can't possibly make enough. That and you barely respond to it at all.[4]

This is where diets like Atkins, and now the Paleo really are a step in the right direction. They cure metabolic syndrome. Take away the wheat and sugar and the problem clears up— sometimes almost immediately. If you've had diabetes for a long time, it may take longer. This shows the body's amazing ability to heal itself. Virtually anything can be regenerated. That's why age reversal works. Just stop abusing the machine and it will fix itself. How cool is that?[5]

The Paleo Diet, which says not to eat anything our ancestors didn't have during the Paleolithic period 10,000 years ago, has enjoyed a lot of popularity lately. It takes away the dairy as well as the flour products. Trouble is it keeps the meat, but tells you to only eat wild caught fish and grass fed beef, etc. too bad. I'm going with what I'll call the "Garden of Eden" diet.

There is a new conventional wisdom emerging and none too soon. It seems we've all been led down a very wrong road (again). For the past 30 or so years, we've been told fat was bad and carbs were good.

There have been several books in recent years elucidating on this notion. Some of the better ones are "Wheat Belly" and "Grain Brain." Doctors wrote these, so you can see this is not radical stuff anymore. These authors are hipping us to the fact that the brain loves fat. The body too needs it to live. Fat is not the enemy. These people, while helping turn the wrong information on fat into the new conventional wisdom, are advocating eating animal fat as well as the healthy kind found in nuts, seeds, avocados, olive oil, etc. We can learn a lot from them without swallowing their message whole.[6]

Wheat is also implicated in degenerative joint issues such as osteoarthritis, and the inflammation it causes. Many people who ditched the wheat have found their joint issues cure themselves. Miraculous? Not at all. Take away the cause and the symptom disappears. Who knew wheat caused so many adverse conditions in the body? Not enough people evidently. The word is slowly leaking out, and many joints as well as waistlines will be the better for it.

A quote from "Wheat Belly": What if, rather than a total hip or knee replacement at age sixty-two; you opted for a total wheat replacement instead? The broader health effects of disrupted acid-base balance are only starting to be appreciated. Anyone who has taken a basic chemistry class understands that pH is a powerful factor in determining how chemical reactions proceed. A small shift in pH can have a profound influence on the balance of a reaction. The same holds true in the human body. "Healthy whole grains" are the cause for much of the acid-heavy nature of the modern diet. Beyond bone health, emerging experiences suggest that crafting a diet that favors alkaline foods has the potential to reduce age-related muscle wasting, kidney stones, salt-sensitive hypertension, infertility, and kidney disease."

We are now seeing "wheat replacement", as Dr. Davis so aptly put it, is an important key to ridding ourselves of osteoarthritis—and a host of other conditions as well. Just be careful not to replace one evil with another. When we cut out all animal "foods", wheat, and soy, we will have room in our lives (and our stomachs) for the foods that will age us in reverse and eradicate disease. Once again, these are vegetables, seeds, nuts, fruit, mushrooms, onions, seaweed, beans, and lots of salad.

We can have a diet that supplies sufficient fat without poisoning ourselves with all the toxins that meat is laden with and clogging up all our systems with gooey dairy and congealed chicken embryos. The news that cholesterol is not the enemy, while no longer a fringe notion, is far from mainstream. Most docs are still fixated on your cholesterol numbers as the end-all, be-all measure of heart disease risk. If your number looks high, they'll put you on statin drugs, which have a host of side effects too numerous to mention here. Statin drugs do not block the absorption of cholesterol from food. They only block the body's ability to make its own, which means it blocks the production of HDL, the "good" cholesterol as well as LDL, the "bad" cholesterol.

A recently appreciated problem with statins is that while blocking the body's production of cholesterol, they also block the pathways by which testosterone, serotonin, CoQ10 and other beneficial substances are made. This is why in Canada statins have to carry a warning on the label stating that taking this drug will deplete CoQ10, and that supplementing CoQ10 is advised. Since CoQ10 is so needed by the heart and circulatory system, and that most people are already deficient in it, lack of such labeling here is one of FDA's dirtiest tricks. The people who need CoQ10 the most are denied this vital bit of information.[7]

Here again, we must educate ourselves. Don't rely on the 'experts' to tell you what works and what doesn't, what is good for you and what isn't. I guarantee that if you try the high fat, low carbohydrate diet advocated by these writers, you would feel heavy and tired even though you might lose weight. This is all another incarnation of the Atkins diet from the 70s. It works to lose weight, but is not healthy in the long run due to all the toxins and artery clogging fat. It is also way too high in protein, which as you'll recall is so detrimental to your bones due to the calcium leaching which occurs when the body tries to bring the blood into a near neutral ph. If you cut the carbs and increase the good fat, you will feel something comparatively few people have ever felt.

I had a friend who swore the Atkins diet made him feel fantastic while at the same time losing weight. Losing weight always feels good unless you're detoxing too fast at the same time. One reason eating the heavy protein characteristic of the Atkins diet made him feel good was that for the first time in his life he was actually digesting this protein because he wasn't eating it with bread or other starch. (More on this later) Taking away the bread is a huge deal. This in and of itself will slow the aging process considerably. The problem with the Atkins diet and the newly named Paleo diet is that they are heavy on the wrong kind of fat and will fill your body full of toxins even though the Paleo diet advocates only grass fed beef, free-range chicken, and wild caught fish.

Fasting glucose level is showing itself to be a very important lab value. In other words—a predictor of disease. Most people's fasting glucose levels are excessively high. Getting the wheat out of your diet will go a long way towards lowering yours. Cinnamon is finding appreciation as a stabilizer of blood sugar.[8]

There is a movie about sugar called "Fed Up." In Atlanta, it played in one theater. The reason only one theater showed it, may relate to partnerships existing between the theaters and companies unflatteringly portrayed in the film, like soft drink and candy manufacturers. This movie shows their products to be very unhealthy indeed. I said at the beginning of this book, that I was not going to try to get you off soft drinks or cigarettes, so I'll let you do your own research if you're not convinced these are beyond bad.

The movie portrays sugar as the new tobacco. The companies that sell all these sugary 'foods' to us and more tragically our kids, are denying that there is a problem with their products just like tobacco companies once did. They even say sugar is not that bad in moderation. Sugar certainly is that bad in any amount, causing an inflammatory cascade of events in the body for which it has no defense.. Again, I am going to assume you are not eating sugar, but are like hopefully all of my target audience, hip enough to know that smoking and sugar are killers.[9]

The American diabetes Association (ADA) stated recently 86% of Americans are pre-diabetic, in other words they have metabolic syndrome, also known as syndrome X, that 29% of Americans have full blown diabetes, and 8% have diabetes but don't know it. Fasting glucose levels in the blood, and blood insulin levels are starting to be recognized as important risk factors—as important as high cholesterol and triglyceride levels. High blood sugar could almost be called the "new" cholesterol.

Healthy sweeteners like honey, maple syrup, and even fruit juice can cause high blood sugar and blood sugar spikes. So how can we sweeten up foods and drinks without causing problems? Try Stevia. Stevia is a South American herb that comes in liquid form ready to use in any recipe. If you taste the liquid form, it doesn't taste very sweet, but when added to food and drinks, Stevia imparts a very nice sweetness. It is also purported to have several health benefits as well.[10] Another I have heard of his xylitol. I haven't experimented with this one, and don't know exactly what it is but I've read that it's a healthy sweetener with no downside.

In case you are ever tempted try artificial sweeteners, or if you already use those, please do some research into what these do to your health. Some are carcinogens. All of them fool your body into craving more sweets. They send a message to your brain that sweetness is coming, but no real sugar ever arrives.

This causes you to crave sugar even more. I hope that you never consume this poison anyway.[11]

I'm writing this to people who are highly motivated to make positive changes but lack the information to make the ones that will actually get them the results they want. Like for instance 'healthy whole grains'. You may be eating whole wheat bread thinking it's better for you than white bread. It's not. All the press that sugar is now getting, being called the new tobacco and all, is wonderful, but a worse menace to health (wheat) goes unreported, unless you get your hands on one of the aforementioned books.

Yes, wheat is worse than even sugar. Why? The main reason sugar is so bad is not that it has nothing but empty calories that make you fat. Actually, there is nothing empty about these calories. They pack some serious heat. Wheat packs even more. One reason sugar is so bad is that it starts this inflammatory fire (blood sugar spikes) which your body tries to put out, but has evolved no mechanism for doing so. Wheat is worse because it packs a different kind of sugar than table sugar. Actually, table sugar (sucrose) only becomes sugar when it is digested. It is a disaccharide, meaning it is comprised of a sugar molecule called fructose and one called glucose. These must be converted into glycogen to be used as fuel.

The sugar in wheat is a monosaccharide - glucose. Table sugar has to be digested through two separate pathways, the gut and the liver, so it takes longer to digest and release into the blood. These are converted into glucose. The sugar in wheat arrives fast and fully loaded to do its damage. This is measured by the glycemic index. The glycemic index is a measure of how fast a food or substance is converted into glucose. Table sugar scores a very high 62, wheat an even more damaging 88. Similarly to the way too much protein causes an acid condition in your blood, which your body must respond to in any way it can to keep you alive, these blood sugar spikes must be dealt with damn the consequences to the rest of the body.[12]

Since we never evolved a defense against these spikes, the body dumps insulin into the blood to quell these blood sugar surges. Insulin is not very efficient at this though, and over time, the insulin receptors actually shut down; more insulin must be made and secreted by the poor overworked pancreas, which may help explain why pancreatic cancer is on the rise. You end up with very high levels of insulin in your blood. Insulin has other functions. Its main function has not evolved to be cleaning up the inflammatory mess caused by the wrong kind of carbs. Insulin's main function is to help the body store energy for lean times. You see, the body is very efficient at storing fat, or hadn't you noticed?

Remember almost no human in history or pre-history ate every day. The body became very efficient at storing calories that were not immediately needed for energy as fat. Insulin's main function is to shuttle glucose into the fat cells. We have a situation where the insulin receptors partially shut down. Massive amounts of insulin are circulating almost all the time, and not being picked up. When you have this condition, and you almost certainly do some degree, you have the newly termed "metabolic syndrome", also known as "syndrome X" or "pre-diabetes". Just about all adults have it; and now a huge percentage of kids have it.[13]

It's been recently shown that children develop it more easily than adults. It's also known as insulin resistance. The next stop on this soon to be wrecked train ride is type-two diabetes. This used to be called adult onset diabetes to distinguish it from type-one kids are born with. Now, so many kids are developing type-two that it is not called adult onset diabetes as much, but more commonly referred to as diabesity.

When you have metabolic syndrome, your body has become a fat storing machine. All this excess insulin causes circulating glycogen (as ATP), your fuel, to be shuttled into your fat cells, whether it's needed for energy or not.

Think about this for a moment. You feel tired and are getting fatter and fatter. Your energy stores are being hijacked. Even if you are not that fat (yet), you are storing fat in preference to burning it as energy; this helps explain why we tend to store more fat as we get older (Your energy-delivery system is working less and less well). You may have heard an obese person tell you they don't eat any more than anyone else does. You probably didn't believe them. Some even eat decidedly less than most folks, yet they continue to put on more fat. This also explains why they have so little energy. You thought they were tired from carrying all that fat around. No. They are living in service to their fat. It's as if the fat has become a parasite.

This also helps explain why "calorie in, calorie out" doesn't work when you have metabolic syndrome. Many people exercise vigorously, cut way down on calories, and continue to put on fat. Some give up and resign themselves to gaining weight. Since carrying extra weight is so detrimental to health, this is a tragic conclusion to draw. Curing metabolic syndrome by cutting out wheat and sugar—or wheat AS sugar is now known to be possible and certain. Get rid of the cause and the effect vanishes.

It's been said that your morning bowl of cereal—even if it contains no added sugar might as well be a hot fudge sundae or candy bar. Starches become sugar. Sugar causes metabolic syndrome. Sugar comes in many forms. The worst of its disguises is "healthy whole grains". Try a smoothie for breakfast instead.

Not all people have metabolic syndrome. Most do to at least some degree. Real adherents to the Paleo Diet or the old school Atkins diet don't. Why? Because wheat and sugar cause it and these diets don't allow wheat or sugar. What this means is that you can cure metabolic syndrome by getting the wheat out. You will probably cure your arthritis too.[14] Undoubtedly, you will lose weight and feel great. Just don't replace one evil with another. We can have a non-toxic Paleo Diet; I like to call it the Garden of Eden diet. Maybe we'll call it garden of eatin diet. We can get our fat from foods that help the body become more vibrant instead of filling it with toxic residue.

We've all heard the term "gluten free", it is seen it on different packaged foods. Gluten is a protein found in wheat. It is largely responsible for the damage wheat does. Wheat is not the only food that contains gluten. We must also avoid spelt, kamut, triticale, barley, and buckwheat. Even oats have some.[15] Oatmeal is touted nowadays as a great breakfast food. Certainly, it is better than bacon and eggs, but with its gluten load and its sticky consistency, it is not what I would want first thing in the morning. We want to get the bowels moving in the morning, not gum the body up with a bunch of sticky, gooey bulk. A blender drink is a much healthier option.

Healthy whole grains do exist. They include amaranth, quinoa, and rice, especially wild rice. I read recently that black wild rice has more antioxidants than blueberries. I don't know this to be true, but it sounds pretty good; Time for a bit of experimentation.

To say that gluten is digestively challenging would be a supreme understatement. The protein structure of gluten is like a matrix of long interlinked fibers that curl in on themselves. This structure prevents digestive enzymes from getting to them effectively. When partially digested gluten makes it into the gut of someone with celiac disease, the immune system mistakes the intact proteins for invaders and unleashes an attack. Even in someone without celiac disease or even what's been called "gluten sensitivity", damage is done by consuming this unnatural food.[16]

In "Wheat Belly," there is a chapter entitled "Dropping Acid," which alerts us to the fact that like animal foods, wheat lowers pH in the body, setting the stage for calcium leaching from bone, and creating an environment favorable to pathogenic attack. An acid pH in the blood has implications in cancer formation and many other disease systems. This acid will not make us see colors or try to stop the war – this acid will kill us. Dr. Davis has done a great job with "Wheat Belly." It's not only informative, but also entertaining. I hope he doesn't take offense with Dr. Fuhrman or me for faulting him on his lack of wisdom as to the dangers of meat and dairy. Perhaps one day, he will see the light. Maybe his next book will be called something like "Meat Heart."

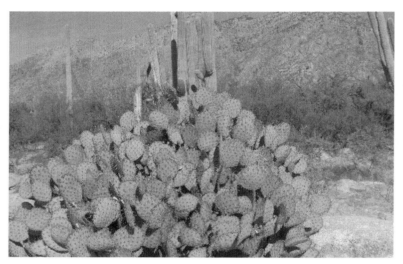

Purple Prickly Pear Cactus in Tucson, Arizona

"Don't worry, be happy."

- Meher Baba

CHAPTER 7
NO JOY IN SOY

A h yes, the soy; It's not the health food it's made out to be. It's not even good for you. One of the great tragedies of our time is that people who are motivated to attain better health through quitting meat and dairy, are often substituting these with soy products. Please don't let this happen to you. Some have even suffered seemingly irreversible effects. Again, I say once you stop an irritant your body will begin to heal itself.

Soy, even if it is organic, is one of the most genetically modified foods we have. Peanuts also have no place in a healthy diet. Corn could join that list as well. These are common allergens. Many people are allergic to soy and/or peanuts. Most of us are allergic to these things. We are not clinically allergic, which means there are no symptoms, yet they are attacking our immune systems just the same. This has caused untold suffering to those who are trying to do better by their health by giving up one evil for another.[1]

There is starting to be quite a lot of information about how bad soy is. Many health professionals advise eating less. I of course say, if its crap leave it alone. Many of the people who have experienced serious health complications from soy, have done so by consuming what one writer has dubbed "frankenfoods." Frankenfoods are highly processed soy products made to look like, and have the texture of meat, bacon, turkey, etc. These are often heated to very high temperatures, which causes runaway glycation.[2] There is an excellent book called "The Whole Soy Story," which shares some of these tragic stories. Like the books on the evils of wheat, I mentioned earlier, this writer advocates meat consumption. We can learn a lot from what these authors have to tell us, without swallowing their message whole. I predict that one-day soy will be widely known to be the enemy of health it is. Until then, we must educate ourselves. Ignorance is anything but bliss.

Soy is just about the cheapest food to grow. It grows abundantly in poor soil, and is very hardy. It is planted at a rapid rate in what was tropical rainforest, to be used mostly in China as animal feed. When they grow it organically here, it becomes a marketer's dream. The profits made on soy rival that of just about any crop out there. Now it's even more profitable because it's GMO—a genetically modified organism. This makes it drought resistant, but like any modified plant, it's much more harmful to your body.[3]

Wheat has had a similar series of modifications. The most modified plant may well be corn. Corn comes from South America. It was a small seed head from a grass similar to wheat. It was smaller than that baby corn used in Chinese food. Through years of modification, we have a grain that seems like a vegetable. Wheat is a far cry from its original form too. The four-foot sheaves that used to be the wheat crop have been reduced to an 18-inch dwarf variety, engineered to be hardy and drought resistant.[4]

Getting back to soy, it was always poison—literally. It, even in its non-GMO form, contains an aflatoxin,[5] which causes stomach cancer among other conditions. I, being the experimenter that I am, and not knowing any better, tried drinking a lot of soy milk in the early 2000's. It filled my body with phlegm, which took years to clear out. Dairy milk also has a ton. Some call it mucous, but it's more properly known as catarrh or phlegm. This stuff forms the perfect breeding ground for nasty organisms.

I read that in 1996 2% of soybeans were modified to be Roundup tolerant, 90% by 2002. Roundup, in case you don't know, is the trade name for a very toxic defoliant. It is used on fields to get rid of weeds.[6] Normally it would kill whatever crop it fell on as well. Therefore, they genetically modify (GMO) the crop to withstand this chemical. I have used Roundup in my yard. It is incredibly potent. If you get a little on the grass instead of the weed you are trying to kill, that spot of grass is done for at least the rest of the season. Any organism that can withstand Roundup is highly modified indeed. I have heard that in America unlike most of the rest of the world, food can be labeled organic even if it is GMO. GMO foods also are not required to carry any sort of labeling stating it is a GMO food.

My challenge in writing this chapter on the evils of soy is to keep it short enough. There is so much to tell it would take a book. That book runs 450+ pages. It's called "The Whole Soy Story" and if I don't succeed in motivating you to give up all soy products, I hope you'll read this book.

Consider lysinoalanine, the cross-linked amino acid produced when lysine, one of the eight essential amino acids, is subjected to alkaline treatments. The soy industry uses alkali to turn soybeans into soymilk, tofu, and textured vegetable protein (TVP), also known as textured soy protein. This is what comprises many vegetarian burgers.[7] Rats fed soy protein have suffered kidney lesions and kidney stones. Iron levels in rats fed soy protein dropped to half of those of controls while copper levels increased threefold. Health professionals generally overlook copper toxicity.[8] It is usually accompanied by a zinc deficiency.[9] Zinc deficiency has been linked to a host of health challenges including depression and anxiety, as well as, diabetes and rheumatoid arthritis.

Excitotoxins are amino acids such as glutamate and aspartate, which are created when food processors hydrolyze soy protein to make hydrolyzed vegetable protein (HVP) and soy sauce.[10] MSG (monosodium glutamate) is a flavor enhancer and can legally be called "natural flavor." Look out for this! It is added to many foods and even juices that would otherwise be healthy. Actually, the term "natural flavors" can legally be used to disguise anything from MSG to beef fat. Not that "natural flavors" are necessarily either one of these, but we don't know.[11] So much for "all natural" prepared foods. What problems can excitotoxins cause in our bodies? Who knows? So many toxins are new. We simply don't know what they can do to us. Don't be a guinea pig.

Broiling, frying, barbecuing, industrial heat processing extrusion and pyrolysis confer potent mutagenic and carcinogenic compounds known as heterocyclic amines (HCAs).[12] In laboratory animals, the organ most vulnerable to HCAs is the liver. Your liver is your largest internal organ carrying out numerous functions. It is not something you can live without. Maybe that is why they call it the live-er. Lung and stomach tumors, lymphomas, and leukemia also occur because of this major health nuisance. Still think your potato chips are an innocent little indulgence? Think again. The higher the heat and the longer the duration, the worse and the more HCAs form. Because modern soy products such as TVP undergo high heat processing, they can carry very high levels of HCAs. Cured meats, such as bacon, sausage, and lunchmeats pose a similar hazard.

Organic solvents such as acetone, benzene, chloroform, cyclohexane, and ether are used to extract oil from beans and seeds.[13] Your so-called "natural" cooking oil could be poisoning you. Certainly your skim milk is. How do you think they skim it? A chemical solvent called hexane. What about decaffeinated coffee? Yep, chemical solvents. What we don't know can hurt us, and does on a daily basis.

One reason for soy's reputation as a health food is that it represents the only complete protein in the vegetable kingdom. As we know now, a complete protein is not necessary in the body, and from a metabolic standpoint is not even possible. Soy is barely a complete protein, meaning that some of the eight amino acids that have to be present for a protein to be considered complete are very poorly represented. The sulfur containing amino acids like methionine are in short supply; not that this really matters.

What does matter is that soy has a protease inhibitor. This prevents the absorption of many amino acids.[14] Protease inhibitors are known to cause thickening of tissues. This contributes to the darkening and hardening characteristic of aging tissues of all kinds.

This is a quote from "The Whole Soy Story": "Whenever protease inhibitors cause cell proliferation (hyperplasia), cancer becomes a distinct possibility. Rapidly growing tissue are more susceptible to chemical carcinogens. Rats exposed to moderate levels of protease inhibitors in raw soy flour show increased susceptibility to cancer, while those subjected to high levels of the inhibitors suffer pancreatic cancer. Trypsin inhibitors potentiate two known pancreatic carcinogens, azaserine, and nitrosamine.[15] Though azaserine is more likely to be found in the laboratory than in the average diet, nitrosamine is a byproduct of food processing found in most modern soybean products. Cancer also occurs in soy fed animals that have not been exposed to known carcinogens."

Phytates are another problem that soy consumption poses.[16] These cause mineral deficiencies and could explain why vegetarians are sometimes low in iron. Some vegetarians can even become anemic; which their friends may immediately jump on, and tell them they'd better eat some red meat before it's too late. Soymilk is often fortified with calcium, as with orange juice and other foods fortified with calcium, it's usually the wrong kind: calcium carbonate and calcium phosphate. The soy industry is trying to give you an alternative to cow's milk. The problem is that the calcium is the wrong kind and the phytates impede the absorption of not only calcium and iron but other minerals as well.

Like the oxalic acid found in spinach, these phytates block the absorption of all the minerals consumed in the same meal. When it comes to a mineral like zinc, which is involved in so many body functions, and is in such short supply in most diets, this is a big deal. Infants fed on soy formula can even die from these mineral deficiencies.

You might think edamame is better because the soybeans are lightly processed, only cooked, and then refrigerated. Yes, anything less processed and less cooked is going to be better. However, Soy in any form contains many anti-nutrients like lectins and saponins.[17] Saponins cause damage to the jejunum, the middle stage of the small intestine where most digestion occurs. There's even an anti-nutrient called Soyatoxin.[18] This causes blood clotting, which can be a very bad thing, leading to phlebitis and stroke. Thick blood is not what we want. The reason some doctors advise folks to take low-dose aspirin every day is to thin the blood.

Another quote from "The Whole Soy Story," Soyatoxin has proved lethal to mice, causing breathing difficulties, convulsions, and partial paralysis prior to death. Lectin induced cell deaths lead to increased cell turnover and a greatly increased requirement for protein needed for DNA and RNA synthesis. The intestinal villi shrank from the combination of premature cell death and replacement by immature cells, changes that alter both form and function. Meanwhile, the deeper so-called 'crypt cells' speed up the production of new cells, producing them at such a prodigious rate that hyperplasia (thickening of tissues) results. As a result, the wall of the small intestine thickens and the organ gains weight. Enlargement of the pancreas may also occur, a condition generally blamed on protease inhibitors but strong evidence suggests that lectins should share the blame."

So, here we are, eating something that causes damage to the small intestine—the organ that digests our food; Not a good plan. Since cancer is a disease characterized by rapidly growing cells and pancreatic cancer is on the rise, we should err on the side of caution and not eat any soy. Ever.

Another anti-nutrient soy delivers is oxalate, also known as oxalic acid. Oxalates bind with calcium and other minerals preventing their absorption. Spinach, rhubarb, and peanuts are also sources. Oxalates play a major role in the formation of kidney stones. Free oxalates can also be absorbed through the intestinal wall into the blood stream. Oxalate is an irritant that causes the release of histamine. Histamine, as part of your immune system, is released when the body perceives a threat. There are whole books written on the dangers of oxalates.[19] A close friend of mine loves peanut butter. He recently underwent surgery to remove kidney stones.

Soy's reputation as a health food is largely based on its content of isoflavones.[20] These have been purported to protect against heart disease and cancer. I wish this were true. I rather like bringing you the news that animal "foods" are killers. I like the fact the foods that cause such suffering to our fellow creatures and our planet cause suffering in us. There is a certain karmic justice in this. If something as cheap and readily available as soy really were beneficial, I would be the first to laud it. Soy though, unfortunately is not something we want to consume.

A quote from "The Whole Soy Story": "the FDA allows products containing soy protein to carry a claim stating that they protect against heart disease. However, the isoflavone genistein, the principal isoflavone in soy protein, can cause heart arrhythmias. Researchers have found that genistein interferes with potassium in the heart, suggesting the potential for soy isoflavones to cause heart arrhythmias."

Here's another quote: "From 1991 to 1993 Lon R. White M.D., a neuro-epidemiologist with the Pacific health Institute in Honolulu, and his team completed cognitive testing on 3734 men, MRI on 574, and autopsies on 290. They analyzed cognitive test data for 502 wives on the assumption that they had eaten the same meals as their husbands. The results? Men and women who ate tofu at least twice per week experienced accelerated brain aging, diminished cognitive ability and were more than twice as likely to be clinically diagnosed with Alzheimer's disease. MRI scans showed enlarged ventricles (in the heart) while autopsies revealed atrophied brains with lower weights. Subjectively, the researchers couldn't help but notice that by age 75 to 80 the tofu eaters looked about five years older than those who abstained."

Soy consumption also negatively effects the thyroid, a small butterfly shaped gland in the front of your neck, which regulates many body functions far out of proportion to its size. Plant estrogens, especially the isoflavones genistein and daidzein are potent inhibitors of thyroid hormones T3 and T4.[21] Low production of thyroid hormone is a huge factor in lack of thyroid function. Large numbers of people in the modern world have malfunctioning thyroid glands due to low thyroid hormone. Iodine, the main nutrient needed by the thyroid, so lacking in the modern diet, does not protect against this effect. In other words even if you have sufficient iodine these isoflavones will inhibit the production of thyroid hormone. The thyroid is not something you want to mess with.

Many of the accounts in "The Whole Soy Story" of people who have been harmed by soy consumption have to do with damage to the thyroid.

Soy is a huge moneymaker for the soy foods industry. It is very cheap to grow and has now been hyped with health giving qualities it never had. When you have enough money you can even get the government stamp of approval apparently. The FDA actually allows soy foods to carry labeling stating health benefits. Don't fall for this. Do your own research if I haven't convinced you that soy is beyond bad. Soy is generally not as much of a health concern as wheat because so few people eat it compared to wheat. At most risk are people who are concerned about their health enough to quit or cut down on animal products, and feel the need for replacement.

When we hear things over and over, we tend to believe them sooner or later. Big business is all over this. Why do you think you see the same commercials repeatedly? We hear the same messages said in so many different ways. Sooner or later, we start to believe what these messages tell us. It's as if the more people repeat things the truer they get. There is so much more I could have written about soy.

I hope if you have always heard that soy is so wonderful, and are having trouble letting go of that notion, that you will do your own research. Please don't do that research by eating soy products—they are far too dangerous.

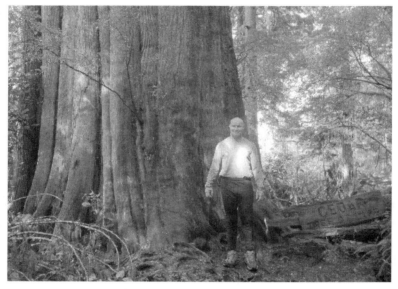

Cedar Tree of Life, Big Tree Trail, Meares Island, Tofino

"Sometimes letting things go is an act of far greater power than defending or hanging on."

- Eckhart Tolle

CHAPTER 8

SPIRITUALITY AND AGE-REVERSAL

R eversing your age is also the greatest gift you can give to humanity. How's that? We are all connected. As you evolve your consciousness, you impart expansion to everyone on the planet. This is what we need to make the change necessary to save ourselves from extinction. I laugh when I hear people talk about saving the planet. The planet doesn't care if we populate ourselves into oblivion. We could even take most other species with us and the earth would just continue without us.

Even the greatest scourge of our, or any other time—nuclear power and weapons - will not matter in the timeline of the earth. I hope we won't let it come to that. It is readily apparent a major shift in consciousness is needed; we have to care more.

Many of us care, but we feel helpless to effect change. We are not. Each one of us has something to say about where this all will go.

I have found as I get cleaner physically, my intuitive centers wake up more and more. My capacity to care about the earth and my fellow beings increases. All my spiritual endeavors are made so much easier. This used to surprise me, as did the fact that there is no end to this. It all keeps getting better and easier. I used to wonder how that was possible. I could understand how the body got stronger and stronger, but why does it make so much difference to how I feel emotionally or spiritually? After all, we are not these bodies these are just "meat suits" we wear for a time. The answer finally came intuitively.

This body is your vehicle. Everything you experience comes through it. The state it's in has everything to do with your soul's evolution, at least while the soul is housed in it.

Another thing that should come as no surprise is that not eating dead flesh and extracted cow goo will make you feel peaceful and calm, as well as energized. There are a few reasons why this is so. When these poor creatures are killed, they're killed on an assembly, or in this case, disassembly line. More than a few observers noticed that after the 2004 tsunami how few animals were killed because they sensed trouble coming and moved to higher ground. Animals have been known to feel earthquakes long before they occur. They obviously have senses we either don't have or have lost. So they probably know well in advance when they are about to be slaughtered. When they are on that disassembly line, seeing and feeling what's happening to the animals in front of them, imagine the fear and horror they are experiencing.

To say they don't feel pain as we do is ridiculous. It sounds to me like what the slave traders and keepers used to say to justify slavery. They said black people didn't feel it when their children were taken from them. That they didn't feel pain in the same way white people do. Someday this crazy way of thinking about animals will be known by anyone with a brain to be just as erroneous.

When you stop eating meat, dairy, fish, and eggs, you remove yourself from this horrible equation. Somehow, we got the idea that some animals matter and some don't. We spend millions caring for our pets, yet treat farm animals with such brutality it defies description. Some cultures worship cows and eat dogs. Some worship dogs and eat cows.

As you get the fear vibration out of your energy field by not eating meat, you will no doubt feel the same. This is why I mention this: when you eat meat, you are also eating fear and adrenalin. The meat is shot full of all that at the time of such a violent end. When you eat their meat, you eat their fear. No wonder everyone is so afraid.

Look what happened after 911.[1] We laid down and allowed our civil rights to be taken away. Fear makes us do dumb things. If you don't know what I'm talking about, Google the so-called "Patriot Act" and see. As you rid your body of the caustic irritant of fear and chemicals so well represented in the meat, you will feel more calm and peaceful than you ever have in your life.

The collective consciousness is expanding at an incredible rate, and one of the more dramatic examples of this is our new understanding of the cause of all disease. No, believe it or not, I'm not talking about toxicity. Toxicity is one of the root causes of cellular degeneration. However, what is now being realized as the root cause of all disease is inflammation. More enlightened doctors (both of them...just kidding) are looking at your c-reactive protein and homocysteine levels as markers of systemic inflammation versus only looking at your LDL cholesterol level as the main risk factor for heart disease. Tragically, this is only done by docs who keep up with the latest research.

This is new knowledge and may not have made it into the med school curriculum yet, and certainly was not when most docs went to school. So most are still hearing alarm bells go off when they see a high LDL number, and prescribe a cholesterol-lowering drug like Lipitor or Crestor. Both have been known for their many side effects.

As we expand our awareness, as we open up more and more to our spiritual side by not consuming dead flesh, our intuitive centers open up. As we listen to our intuitive guidance, we choose to be guided. When we choose to be guided by our intuition, its voice becomes louder and clearer. We must listen to our intuition especially when it comes to our health. We cannot rely on medical professionals to tell us what we need. They are products of their training. Sometimes, their training is severely lacking in addressing the causes of the symptoms we are experiencing. Sometimes we have no symptoms, yet we allow these professionals to prescribe something our intuition tells us we do not need.

Case in point: I once had a massage client who came to me seeking relief for a muscle wasting disease his doc called polymyositis.[2] This is a condition whereby the muscles atrophy at a phenomenal rate and hurt all the time. He was a healthy 30-something at the time, who went in for a routine checkup. His doc saw a higher LDL number than he wanted to see and so prescribed Lipitor. My client refused to take it as he'd heard some horror stories about the stuff. His doc insisted that he take something to lower his LDL number. He finally agreed to take Crestor, which he was assured was safer. Within days of starting it, he had severe pain all over his body and was weak and very tired. When he called the doc to tell him of this vexatious turn of events, he was told to stop the med, and cautioned not to exercise in an attempt to slow the muscle wasting, as this would cause the pain to become even more severe.

He was not inclined to follow this doc's advice anymore and so tried to work out. He found out that the doc did know something. He was right about the pain from working out. The doctor could not offer any treatment for the disease the Crestor caused but only advised him to stop taking it. His doctor and other docs he saw subsequently said that while his new disease had a name, it did not have a cure. It was known to be an uncommon side effect of Crestor.[3] It would hopefully get better now that he had stopped taking the drug. He had only taken the drug a few days, and now has a condition with no cure that robs him of his muscle. To my knowledge, it never did improve.

We all know people with similar stories. This guy was healthy before his checkup. In doing research on his condition, I found this quote: "Statins can cause the immune system to attack the muscles and other body systems." The take-home message is; clean up your diet and you won't have to risk the side effects of any drug.

What can we learn from his experience? Follow your own "inner knowing" springs to mind. Educate yourself, is certainly another. Do your research and follow your gut. These cholesterol numbers are set quite arbitrarily and don't allow for any variation. For example, the numbers they consider in the normal range for cholesterol don't allow for the fact some people make more than others do naturally. These drugs do not stop your body from absorbing cholesterol from your food. They stop your body's manufacture of cholesterol. Often, the docs we trust with our most prized possession are not giving us any other alternative but to go on drugs. If you stop eating the animal fat, your cholesterol will drop on its own. Even eating less will help. Remember, though, to age in reverse you have to stop all animal fat.

This man had a very clear message from his intuition that the statin drugs were not something he needed, and could harm him. He went against his inner knowing, deferring to the doctor who insisted he take them. As you clean the fear vibration from your consciousness by stopping the consumption of dead flesh, your intuitive centers will open up to a degree that will amaze you. As you honor its guidance by allowing yourself to be guided, you will get more and more intuitive input. In other words, by listening to your inner knowing, you are inviting and embracing your intuition. You will also save yourself a lot of trouble!

An often feared and very widely discussed symptom of aging is brain fog, dementia, Alzheimer's and senility. Let me state here that these conditions are no more a natural part of the aging process than ADD and ADHD are a natural part of childhood. The same thing of course causes them. No, not genetics. Lifestyle. Lots of new research to share on this subject.

First, the most exciting, this is new stuff, so as with much new research, it contradicts the old and still widely held beliefs. Here it is. Brain cells can regenerate.[4] If that doesn't seem earth shaking to you, let me show you why this is an absolutely game-changing finding. It was thought that you were born with a set number of brain cells and that unlike the rest of the body, which renews cells on a daily basis, once brain and nerve cells are dead they are dead, and no new ones will be regrown or regenerated. It has long been known, for example, that one alcoholic drink kills upwards of a million brain cells. Other drugs kill brain cells too.

I'm not suggesting the news that brain cells are regenerated is good news because now that you know you can grow more brain cells you can do drugs and alcohol. When you get the buzz of super-health and unlimited energy, you won't want drugs. They will only diminish the wonderful high you have going on. The reason it's such good news is that age reversal is all about regeneration of cells. If there were really a body part that was out of our ability to influence, our efforts to regenerate would be limited. Now we know there is no part of the body that cannot be regenerated. No more excuses. Let's do this.

Why does the brain age at such an accelerated rate anyway? We know that it does and that this rate is accelerating. All symptoms of brain aging are on the rise, and not because we have so many old folks about now. We baby boomers will soon be joining their ranks. No, this Alzheimer's (old-timer's) stuff is new, as is ADD and ADHD. Did we hear about them when we were kids?[5]

It's like how people at the turn of the last century weren't hearing about cancer and heart disease. This is not because people didn't live long enough to get these diseases. Cancer is a relatively new phenomenon.[6] In the last few years, colon cancer has risen to number three on the cause of death list in America. These symptoms of aging are on the rise, there can be no debate about that.

Back to the question of why the brain, along with the rest of the body is aging so fast. First of all, the brain uses some 20% of the body's oxygen.[7] How does it get all this oxygen? From the blood. Stroke occurs when the supply of blood to one or more areas of the brain is diminished even a little, even if it's only for a few seconds. This can result in permanent paralysis to one or more parts of the body depending on how severe the blockage was and where it occurred. Stroke is also a major cause of death in developed countries where we eat lots of foods that supply the material to clog, fully or partially, these pathways. Our brains are under the same sorts of attacks as the rest of our bodies, but are far more sensitive to them.

We live in fear of these neurological disorders like Alzheimer's. Many of us fear this type of aging most of all. For good reason it seems. It and all the other feared symptoms of cognitive decline are on the increase. Again, I say this is not because there are a greater number of older people now. This, like all diseases or symptoms of aging, is steadily increasing. Some, like Alzheimer's and colon cancer appear to be racing up the charts. Fortunately, the fix is the same for all of them, stop eating junk. Don't fear them, because the law of attraction states that you get what you fear. Don't put your mental energy into that which you don't want. It's been said that worry is misuse of imagination.

Since I broached this subject, allow me to digress for a moment to explain a bit about how this works. Maybe a discussion on the brain is a good time for a little light on this subject. We program our personal reality by the thoughts we think, period. Our subconscious mind is driving our behavior from beneath the level of conscious thought. The media masterminds know all about this. As you connect more and more with the subconscious mind, you will see this more clearly.

The subconscious only listens to here and now statements. It responds to only positive in-the-moment programing.[8] In other words, you can and do program your subconscious with thoughts such as, "I am getting stronger and healthier every day." Not to mean your subconscious doesn't hear negative thoughts, just that they have to be of the here and now variety. Saying, "I hope this doesn't happen" is the same as saying "I hope this happens" to your subconscious. It's very important to feed your subconscious the thoughts you want to see come to fruition. Check out the book or video "The Secret" for more on how the subconscious creates our reality.

Luckily, this is not an instantaneous manifestation. We are allowed as it were, an errant thought, and the thoughts do not, thank God, manifest instantly. When you keep thinking the thought though, it will surely come to pass. This is freewill in action. Understanding how this works is one more step in the direction of being able to use your freewill. As you work with this, you will see how little actual freewill most people have. You will also see how quickly you can re-establish yours. Just knowing you have choices gives you choices.

Just knowing that you have lost contact with the subconscious is enough to start you on the road to freedom. An integrated being is who you are. A free and autonomous entity is what you naturally are. Your soul's native state is complete and absolute freedom. This is why it takes so little effort to get back to it - you're already there. In addition, as we grant freedom to other beings, we get more ourselves. As you do your part to alleviate suffering, your suffering will disappear. Stopping eating meat and dairy is the best way I can think of to do this. Set the slaves free and we will be free.

Ours is a violent society, or hadn't you noticed? We condone violence. I once met a kid who received a ten-year sentence for growing pot. You can beat up your wife and walk away with a warning. We invade other countries at will. We started the arms race. We perpetuate it. We make more and more nuclear waste every day even though there is no way to store it safely. We are leaving it all for our children to deal with. Thank you for allowing me a bit of a rant there. I feel better now.

If you indulged me that far without throwing the book across the room (if you did, you proved my point about our violent society), allow me one more little speculation. Many of us view life not as a one shot deal, but as a series of incarnations..., which explains talents, instant recognition of people or places, Deja vu, etc. I have read widely on this subject, being unsatisfied with the conventional wisdom (imagine that).

The consensus from some highly revered spiritual masters is we tend to incarnate on the same planet repeatedly, and are drawn to the same souls like our immediate family repeatedly, which would help explain why there's often so much drama in families. Soooo, if for example, we leave a world spiked with waste that's radioactive for tens of thousands of years to our descendants, guess what? We are them. If you believe in a literal Hell—well, maybe we are creating it.

We as inhabitants of the industrial world are enjoying a period of unsustainable prosperity. It can't last. We all know that intuitively. There is no time but the present, so let's enjoy it. I think we could be having a lot more fun if we had more concern for our future selves though. I really don't enjoy feeling like part of the problem.

I grasped the enormity of our situation early on and for most of my life, I felt like part of the problem. I felt like just another cog in the machine that is consuming the planet. I finally realized I wasn't. As one of the people who cares about the earth and humanity, I am a vector for change. As someone who aspires to get healthier in every way and do less damage to myself and other beings, I am a positive influence on this so-called reality. This was an amazing revelation. No more am I an angry young man, now I'm a vessel for the light, an example of what's possible. Maybe that's a bit too grandiose, but I'm claiming it.

As we clean up our personal act, we become vectors for change. As Gandhi said, "Be the change you want to see in the world." He also said, "What you do may seem unimportant, but it is most important that you do it." It starts with each one of us. You don't just do age reversal for yourself. You do it for everyone alive, our children, and our future selves. As you expand your consciousness and claim more of your freewill, you put freedom into the mass consciousness. You are part of the solution. We can have this incredibly high standard of living without trashing the planet. All we have to do is be less violent. It starts with what you put into your body.

I know, you bought this book to learn how to reverse the aging process. What's all this hippie crap? As you try the suggestions in this book, you will awaken your compassionate side—your heart. You will become peaceful and calm beyond anything you can now imagine. You will begin to care more and more about things outside yourself. You will become more in tune with things inside yourself. You will find that the kingdom of God is truly inside of you; God is not something "out there". Now, I've really crossed the line. If you don't presently resonate with what I am saying here, just shake your head, call me a new-age creep, and keep reading. I don't care if you agree with me; just don't let anything stop you from having the gift of age reversal. It is a gift that keeps on giving to yourself and everyone else; it is a gift you give yourself. Just so you know, I'm not a hippie, I'm a happie.

Don't take it all too seriously. Many of us have a problem with this. Silly talking monkeys. We take life, in general, way too seriously. In yoga philosophy, this life is known as "Lila"– God's play.[9] The idea is to watch the play, be entertained by the play but not to be caught up in it. God's play is a comedy. If you're not laughing, you're missing the punchline. If you're not having fun here, you're not living. And, if you can't find a way to wring some joy from this life, don't worry; it will be over soon! A big reason why people don't have more fun is they are too damned serious.

I laugh when people call me a strict vegan. If they knew me, they would not refer to me as strict in any sense of the word. I just found something amazing and am in no hurry to mess it up. I'm all about the fun. If this were not fun, I would not do it. If it were a constant battle of wills, I would lose. Willpower stopped being needed many years ago. Once you establish the new pattern, willpower is no longer a vital component of your makeup. Once you feel the difference, you will not be tempted anymore. I look at the stuff people eat; it doesn't look like food to me.

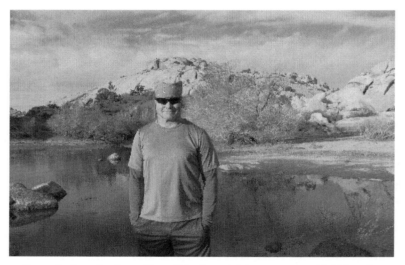

Lost Lake, Joshua Tree National Monument, California

"Courage is the most important of all the virtues because without courage, you can't practice any other virtue consistently."

- Maya Angelou

CHAPTER 9
MUSCLE IS YOUTH

I want to say a bit about the aging face, and how to make it age in reverse. You can regenerate it to an unbelievable degree. What is happening is that at the same time the skin is losing elasticity and cellular water, you are losing muscle mass under it. Remember that after age 25 the average person loses somewhere around a pound of muscle a year.[1] When those small muscles in the face atrophy, there's not as much holding the shape of the face. The neck muscles also get a lot smaller (sarcopenia). Hideous. While this is happening, the skin is drying out.

EFAs (essential fatty acids)[2] are important here, to moisturize your face from the inside. Of course, what moisturizes your face from the inside also moisturizes your internal organs, keeping them supple. This is so very important in your arteries particularly. New research is showing them to be complex organs, not a bunch of tubes. Keeping them supple is one way to prevent occlusion.

Occlusion (full or partial blockage) is what causes stroke and Alzheimer's. When blood flow is partially or fully blocked to one or more parts of the brain, stroke and partial, or full paralysis, is the result.[3]

Back to the face, these muscles do not have to atrophy. All we need to do is to strengthen them. How? Same way you strengthen any muscle. Wooork it. One of the best ways to do this is by performing oral sex. Truly, it is more blessed to give than to receive. Another is isometrics, where you hold tension on the muscles. You can purse your lips together, hold in a straight line (no smile or frown) and flex your facial and neck muscles, being careful not to furrow your brow. Feel the facial muscles flex or watch them in a mirror. Experiment for the experience. It's from the nostrils down that we are primarily working. Engage the neck muscles too.

It's somewhat difficult to describe the facial isometric workout. I find as I try, that it seems to all come from the lips. Squeeze them together in a straight line. Feel the outside corners flex and curl downward. Particularly pay attention to the muscles at the sides of and just below the lips. The small muscles between the mandibles (edge of the jaw) and the chin are the ones we most want to target. You can feel them activating. Keep experimenting, feeling the facial muscles in different ways and at different angles. Practice in front of a mirror. You will be rewarded with a "face lift" that never droops or needs to be re-done.

Do your facelift exercise as you would any workout—you want the muscles to receive enough work to become sore the next day. Then you want to rest them and allow them to recover. You want to overstress them so they are stimulated to grow. Any amount of work you make them do will tone them. To make them grow you have to do enough exercise to make them sore. You can do this isometric workout while driving or watching TV.

Also try what I call neck curls. Laying on a flat surface, you bring your chin to your chest from a supine, (lying on your back) position. Exhale on the upward movement, inhale as you lay the head back down. Keep doing this rhythmically, breathing every repetition. Go for sets of at least 50. Do as many sets as you can. I have done as many as 30 sets of 200. The neck responds to training really fast. You can bring the abdominal muscles into it by keeping your legs raised while you do the neck curls. If you hold them raised, straight up (toes pointing at the sky) you will receive the most abdominal benefit. An easier way is to have them bent (toes pointing opposite your head). Easier still is to have the feet flat on the same surface as the rest of your body. Easiest of all is to have them straight out in the lying down (supine) position.

Another is my "couch potato" exercise. This is good if you can't do the neck curls, due to injury or tightness. If you feel pain in the back of the neck when doing the neck curls, you can do this one and get a similar effect. All you do is lay supine on your back and lift your head up. Use your abdominal muscles like you were starting to do a crunch, but just stay there. The higher you go up, the harder it is. Just hang out in that position. You will feel it in your abs and your neck. I've never found anyone who could not do this exercise. You can just hang out in this position. It's cool to have a TV directly in front of you, to take your mind off what you are doing. Best not to have the neck twisted. Reading in this position also works.

The first time I watched a whole half hour show in this position was cause for celebration. I can do it now for 4 hours or so. When you start to fatigue, your neck may tremble. If you push past this point a bit, you will get the most benefit. Eventually, you will have to lay your head back down. Rest for a few seconds, and come up again. It's like doing sets of weight training, only the weight is your head and shoulders. No strain on your neck can occur. It's all isometric. This exercise trains your entire "core" with no strain on your neck or back. It works your abdominal muscles as well as your neck.

The neck curls are something to aspire to if you can't do them now. They are a bit harder than the couch potato. As I said, if you bring your legs up in the air and hold them either straight up (hardest), or bent during neck curls, you will engage the abdominal muscles as well. Building more muscle in your neck has many benefits. You will not only look younger, you will feel much more vital and energized. If the front of your neck and your abs are sore the next day, that means you will be building muscle. Your neck will be much less susceptible to injury as it becomes stronger.

When we work out, we injure the muscles. We "tear down" the muscle fibers – the catabolic phase. Now is the time to rest and let them recover – the anabolic phase. If you didn't get sore, go harder the next time. Many people make the mistake of working out too often. Best to rest until the muscles fully recover. Now you can trash them again. Each time you do, they will become stronger. Keep in mind that any exercise that builds muscle builds bone as well. Major league baseball pitchers have been shown to have up to 10 times the bone density in their pitching arm than they have in their other arm.

I don't mean to give the impression that we don't want to exercise every day. What I mean is when you get sore from a workout the muscles have been injured. This is a good thing— a very good thing. Now, they must recover to build back stronger and bigger. I have heard people express concern that they will become too big like a bodybuilder from doing this. What a laugh. Do you know how much work it takes to get that big? Relax. Kick your workout and grow stronger.

One of the benefits of training the neck muscles is that by strengthening the front of your neck, you give help and support to the back of the neck, where so many folks have major tension and pain. You have two sets of muscles running the length of your spine to the back of your head. They are the "erectors." They are the ones that hold you up—erect you. When they have to do all the work, they get tired and tense. By strengthening the front of the neck, you give the erectors some much needed help and relief, same with the back muscles. Strengthening the abs will go a long way toward alleviating back pain and strain.

I experienced this in the 80s. I was seriously into mountain biking. Sometimes I would get to the top of a climb and have to throw the bike down and straighten my low back. I was not alone. Low back pain is epidemic in this country and the sedentary affluent societies. I was not sedentary, but I still had a low back issue. Surely having a bit, or a lot, of extra weight in the front doesn't help either. I didn't have that, but my low back still hurt.

In the early 90s, I started white water kayaking, which if you do it right, is a real abdominal workout. I was really into it, and did it every weekend. If my abs had recovered sufficiently from my weekend exertions, I would do some crunches or sit-ups during the week. This all strengthened my abs quite a bit. Lo and behold, my lower back pain vanished, never to return. I have worked with folks who had severe back of neck pain, which has completely disappeared (by doing neck curls). Muscle, as they say, is youth. When you feel the difference, you will want more. Be greedy.

Building muscle throughout the body is a wonderful hobby. Just remember to let the muscles recover between workouts. I do some training with clients. They are amazed when I tell them that I can take them through a complete full-body workout in 15 minutes. The secret is to go to "failure" and slightly beyond on every set.

One of the best moves for building a strong upper body is pushups. Yeah, I know, you can't get down on the floor and push your whole upper body up. That's just like bench-pressing half your body weight, so don't do it on the floor. You can put your hands on the back of a couch, the seat of a chair, a table, or whatever's handy. The lower you go the harder it is. You can even put your hands on the wall for the easiest pushup. Now, you exhale on the upward push. Always exhale when you're doing the working part of the move in any exercise. Get into a rhythm and do some pushups. If your hands are closer together, you bring the chest muscles into it more. Further apart, it becomes more about the front of your shoulders. When you get to the point that you can't do any more, try to bang at least two more. Then...stop at the top of the move and rest for a few seconds. Then do a few more. Body builders know this as ROB, rest only briefly. It allows you to go to "failure" and beyond. Now do something else, like your neck work, and come back for another set of pushups. Two sets should do it.

You see, it doesn't take long, especially at first. You will see how it can all be done in 15 minutes. I don't mean 15 minutes a day either. I mean 15 minutes a WEEK. If you do this well, you have worked the whole body. Now rest.

The other moves, besides neck/ab curls, and pushups, could be squats, which you can do between sets of the other moves. None of this takes any weights or other equipment, but a pair of light dumbbells would be great. You can come up with your own moves as well. Some kind of "military press" is awesome too. This move pushes a weight, or just the weight of your hands, up straight from the shoulders to extend above your head. If you do it with no weight, you will have to do more, but do 50 or so, and you'll feel it. It's great to count and keep a log of the moves you do and the reps you get from week to week. It's fun to see yourself doing more reps every week. Always push for more. Fun. You will feel the difference.

I watched a show on PBS called "The Truth about Exercise", wherein the host had his blood level of cholesterol, glucose, C-reactive protein, etc. etc. checked to see if exercise could have any effect on these levels and how fast that effect could be obtained. He also had his VO2 max checked. He had virtually every diagnostic test known to man. He was then asked to do a work out three times a week consisting of a three-minute warm-up on an exercise bike, followed by one minute at maximum exertion, in other words, flat out– as hard as he could go for one full minute. This was followed by a two minute cool down. Basically, he was asked to work out for 15 minutes a week. Every factor in his blood work improved. LDL cholesterol improved and every other marker and risk factor was reduced dramatically—in just a couple of weeks.

I tried this particular work out and found it to be a bit harder than it sounds. I can easily go 30 seconds flat out, but if I don't have a clock to tell me a minute has gone by, I am never able to do the full minute. I can't say I have experimented too much with this work out because it does stress your legs, so then my mountain bike rides are compromised. It seems like an awesome way to go if you don't get to ride or run very much due to time constraints.

I recently heard of another approach to this high-intensity training (HIT). This way sounds quite a bit easier but still gives you a similar effect I would think. High-intensity training has been shown to be superior to longer efforts done at less intensity. This used to be called interval training, wherein you warm-up, go really hard and then cool down in repeated cycles. The other way, I referenced, is to warm-up then do 30 seconds flat out, then cool down. The recommended workout is seven cycles. Mountain biking, with its short intense efforts to get up hills, and then coasting down replicates this sort of workout. You can, of course, do any ride or run alternating hard and easy efforts. HIT is the way to go for maximum benefit from your workouts. You see? Like strength training done to failure and beyond for short duration, not much time is needed to get major benefits.

A primary benefit of working out is that muscle burns fat. The muscle is vibrant tissue that requires energy to maintain itself. As we age, we put on fat and loose muscle mass (or hadn't you noticed?) Our metabolisms slow down. Why?

Because we lose muscle. Remember, the average person loses somewhere around a pound of muscle a year after age 25. This is called muscle atrophy or sarcopenia.

To visualize the effect of sarcopenia picture a leg, cut off at the mid-thigh. In a 25 year old, you would be looking from where the foot used to be, toward the torso. You would see the thighbone (femur) surrounded by muscle, with a layer of fat just under the skin. In a 45 year old, you would see the same, only the composition would be different. In the older guy, you would be looking at about half muscle and half fat. The size of the leg might not be different, the diameter may even be the same, but aging is happening, atrophy is having its way with the older dude. If the older guy were to work out, run or bike, etc., it would not have to be this way. He could have more muscle and less fat than the young guy.

This, of course is what is happening throughout the entire body. No wonder old folks look like their skin is sagging. The muscle that used to be under it has gone. Sometimes the skin doesn't sag. Sometimes it fills with fat. Yuk. There's no reason for this to happen to you, it probably already has. No worries. Get that muscle back. As you clean up your diet, you will feel more and more like doing this. Just remember to let the muscles recover between workouts. You are not building muscle during a workout, you are tearing it down. You build it during the rest phase while giving it proper nutrients and leaving it alone. I'm talking protein right? No, the average person in industrialized countries already gets too much. I have something even better. NAC (N-acetyl cysteine) helps muscle recover and cures cancer—before it starts.

NAC is a precursor (raw material), or building block of glutathione, which is your body's master antioxidant. The liver produces it, but production slows with advancing age. The liver is unable to make it without the raw material. NAC supplies that raw material.

An antioxidant, as you may know, protects the body from damage by "free radicals", among other insults. It also kills cancer cells. Yes, it cures cancer. You see, we all have cancer. Cells mutate in weird ways due to a whole host of causes. Cancer was rare a hundred years ago. It was thought that was because people didn't live long enough to get it. Now we know that it's on the rise because of toxins in the environment and our consumption of animal products.[4]

So many substances are carcinogenic. It's virtually impossible to avoid exposure to something that causes cancer. Seems now that even our beloved cell phones are on that list.[5] Don't want to give up your phone? Just be sure you keep your immune system healthy, and limit the exposure as best you can by not holding it against your head (use speakerphone) and not wearing it on your body, and not sleeping with it in the same room if possible. Since we can't avoid carcinogens, it makes sense to protect ourselves.

A cell that becomes cancerous must be killed by the immune system. This happens every day. It's a process called "apoptosis"—programmed cell death. You get cancer essentially, and it's cured on the spot—or not. If this cell death does not occur, you really do have cancer. If your immune system is overwhelmed by the volume of carcinogens you are exposed to, or if your immune system is not up to the task, you have a life threatening disease that kills millions of people a year—mostly in developed countries. Fortunately, there are many ways to avoid this.[6]

One is to keep your whole body vibrant and strong. We ingest many carcinogens voluntarily too. I hope that you don't anymore. NAC helps by giving the liver the raw material to make glutathione. In times of stress, both mentally and physically, glutathione is depleted. Glutathione is your body's master antioxidant—many other antioxidants are made from it. It is also depleted by fasting/detoxification, hard exercise, and other stressors. In addition, as you age you make less of it.

I got hip to it by reading an article in Life Extension Foundation magazine. The article described how NAC could cure cancer before it starts.[7] One sentence near the end caught my eye. It said that for athletes it's great because it decreases the soreness caused by heavy workouts, and helps you recover quicker. I thought I could use a bit of that, and noticed NAC was very inexpensive. I ordered some, not expecting much.

I've been reading about, and then using supplements all my adult life. Something like CoQ10, which I'll discuss later, I started taking because it seemed like a good thing with some benefits. I don't expect to feel it. Some people do feel supplements much more, because they are so severely deficient in a nutrient that the difference can be dramatic. Guess I've never been that depleted. The NAC, on the other hand, made a huge difference. I noticed right away that I didn't feel nearly as sore after a workout. I usually take 4 60 mg capsules at a time.

You know that saying, "no pain no gain?" They're not just talking about what you feel while you're working out.

I forgot to mention when I was talking about how little time a full body workout takes that it will hurt a bit. This pain is temporary. It's kind of fun to push through. It may release endorphins, your body's natural painkillers. This can even produce the wonderful "runner's high", along with the joy of pushing through past limitations and expanding our capacity. This accounts, in part, for the addictive nature of exercise. Lotsa fun.

The pain that comes after the exercise and hangs around for days is not as much fun. When it hurts to scratch your nose because your triceps are so hammered from your last workout, it is gratifying, but still hurts. You know you did something good for yourself, but sometimes it's a damned nuisance. NAC to the rescue; Try it. It is an inexpensive supplement.

One more word about working out. I did promise that if you do it right, you can get a whole body workout in 15 minutes. As you get stronger, it will take longer. By then, you will be so into feeling and seeing the wonderful effects that you won't mind more exercise. All you have to do is take it one workout at a time. Just start. Don't say you don't have time. Say...you don't want to. Say...it hurts. Anyone can find time to do this. You can do a set and then do something else like sit at the computer, or vacuum the carpet, then come back for another.

I like to take all day to do my upper body. I'll do a set to failure, then do a chore or sit at the computer for a few minutes, then go hit another. This helps me do max reps on every set. Most body builders do a chest day, then a leg day, etc., working out most days on one or two areas for an hour or so. This is a good way to do it because it keeps your metabolism high and burns fat. It's been known for a decade or so that if you work out in the morning your metabolism is revved up for the whole day. This helps you burn fat all day. I have never done it this way. I've been meaning to try it, but I like it the way I do it, which is to get it all done in one long day.

Some cross-stress occurs when you work a different muscle group. In other words, if you're doing a chest day today, but you already did a back day, you will have to use your arms to do both. Either your arms get hammered again, or you can't go as hard on one of the workouts. You need endurance to do it all in one day though, and most people don't have that kind of endurance. I met a big, super well defined bodybuilder and was telling him how I work out. He said he didn't have the endurance do all muscle groups in the same day. Kinda stroked my ego. That's the idea with the 15-minute workout. You get it all done, and then you rest until the muscles recover (usually about a week for me).

Another way to do it is what's called "circuit training", wherein you do all the moves one after another in quick succession, thereby making an aerobic workout out of it. This also gets it done even faster.

I should say there is another factor in my decision to work all upper body muscles in one day instead of the more conventional approach. I never do legs in the weight room. I tried it, but it messes up my bike riding by making my legs too sore to go hard on riding days.

I am a passionate mountain biker. To me there is nothing better. I do it hardcore at least once a week. This is most definitely not exercise. I differentiate between exercise and a workout. Exercise is great, but a workout is where the idea is to get sore, to trash the muscles so that they build back stronger. This is what I wish for you—you do your strength workout once a week or whatever works for you, but you find a sport that gets you excited. Then it's not a workout at all. It's play. Biking is a pure joy I look forward to all week. As soon as I get off the bike, all hammered and sore, I'm dreaming of the next ride. I hope you can find that kind of passion for something. Some other sports I love are lift-served downhill mountain biking, kayaking, both white water and ocean, playing drums, and backpacking and hiking, particularly in winter.

If you don't have a sport to be passionate about, you don't know what you're missing. Maybe something you used to do when you were younger will be the one as you age in reverse. You will be recapturing your youth in many ways as you stop eating the crap that was killing you. You will do that sport better than you ever used to, I guarantee. We get wiser, hopefully, as we age. We are usually much better off financially, though this may change if we don't do something about runaway inflation. At least your waistline won't be inflating. The kids are grown. It's our time to travel and enjoy life. Tragically, that's when the body starts to feel the effects of our addictions.

Just when we have it made, the body starts to get unmade. The law of entropy states that order becomes disorder. Something not maintained will begin to decay. Don't let this happen to you just when life becomes fun. We always seem to be looking for the next thing. Like the carrot dangled in front of the donkey to keep him moving, we never seem to get there. We say something like "when I retire," "when the weekend comes," "when I meet my soul mate." The future never gets here. This is what's so great about age reversal. It's here and now. It's also really fun.

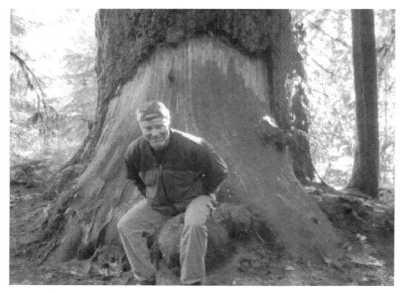

Cathedral Grove, Vancouver Island, British Columbia

"What lies behind us and what lies before us are tiny matters...compared to what lies within us."

- Ralph Waldo Emerson

CHAPTER 10
PROBIOTICS

The word "probiotic" refers to beneficial microbes that inhabit our digestive systems, and indeed every system of our bodies. They are very important to immune function, digestion, and virtually all facets of the body's function. Without them in abundance, the whole body is in a severely compromised position. Building up their numbers and stopping our consumption of the massive amounts of antibiotics in meat and dairy will restore optimal functioning to every part of our bodies. We must restore the body's ecology. We must improve our internal environments. It's been said that the cell is immortal; it's the fluid it lives in that becomes unable to sustain life. In addition, pathogens, viruses, bacteria, fungus, etc. mutate because of the host they land on. Therefore, what is dangerous to one person or animal is not dangerous to another. This explains why two people are exposed to the flu for instance, one gets it, and the other doesn't. One's immune system is working well, the other's isn't. One reason for this is the pathological beds of catarrh, which form the perfect breeding ground for nasty organisms; another is lack of friendly bacteria—probiotics.

The latest research is showing that bacteria make up a huge percentage of your body's weight. If you don't have enough of the good kind to keep the bad kind in check, you compromise the immune system, Sometimes fatally so.

The consumption of alcohol destroys probiotics (as well as brain cells). The massive amounts of antibiotics in meat and dairy kill probiotics off as well. Most people are severely deficient in the beneficial flora so essential to our health.

I read that since the advent of gnomic sequencing that read the DNA in our cells, biologists realized that for every one human cell in our body there are 10 microbial cells. "The idea that we are more microbe than mammal is more profound than the theory of evolution," says a scientist who is involved in mapping the micro biome. The American gut project is devoted to genetically mapping the microbiome. Since the human genome has been mapped now, this seems to be the next frontier in DNA research. Very exciting stuff.

When your personal microbiome is unbalanced, due to too many of the bad guys and not enough of the good guys to keep them from doing their damage, your energy levels and immune system are severely affected. Some of the nation's top scientists go so far as to say that unhealthy microbiomes lie at the heart of the most prevalent health issues today like heart disease, obesity and cancer.

We must replenish our stores of probiotics. We must build up our defense against invasion. We must stop eating substances that kill the beneficial microbes in our digestive tracts and throughout the body. In other words, we must stop eating meat and dairy products, and endeavor to build up a healthy microbial population in our bodies.

I've been doing some reading about mold, particularly black mold.[1] This stuff is not a problem in nature, but when it grows in a building, big trouble can ensue. It needs only moisture and something to live on. Dust will do. Some office buildings have it growing in the ductwork, where it is circulated throughout the building. It will grow just as well on unpainted wood. It seems that 25% of the population is severely affected by this. Some people can go one time into a "sick building," and never be the same. This has been put down to genetics. They say 25% of the population has a genetic weakness to mold. I'll bet further research will show that it's not a genetic weakness at all, but that 25% have such severely compromised immune systems, they are unable to resist the invader when it is inhaled.

It's also been said that kids having a weak immune system causes autism at least in part. Some have been cured of this supposedly incurable disease by building up their probiotics. This is very exciting indeed.

There is a doctor in England whose son was autistic. She was not accepting that his condition could not be improved, so she set out to find what might be missing and causing this condition. She evolved what she called the GAPS diet. GAPS stands for Gut and Psychology Syndrome. Her son was cured completely of his autism through probiotic supplementation. Her practice now is all about working with children who have autism and reversing the condition. She has an excellent book documenting this journey and explaining that probiotics are so severely lacking in modern diets. Her name is Dr. Natasha Campbell Mc Bride. The book is "Gut and Psychology Syndrome". Depression can also be greatly improved or even cured by probiotic supplementation. Some people have even stopped taking anti-depressants after their intestinal flora built up sufficiently.

What does this mean for us age reversers? Only that we need to supplement with probiotics too. You see, every time you eat cooked food, probiotics are destroyed. When you eat raw food, they are replenished. Since most of us eat much more cooked than raw, it makes sense to get some more probiotics in there. This has gone mainstream fast. Now you're even seeing ads for them on TV. The makers of the acidophilus capsules (yogurt culture), say if the probiotic supplement is not refrigerated, it's not alive. The makers of the dry non-refrigerated ones say the opposite. Here again, who do you believe? No one. Grow your own.

I've also found one test for whether a probiotic supplement is working or not is if you burp a little, it is working. Your experimenter, ever working for you, has definitely found the limits. I've done so much I was burping like a man possessed. Guess I was possessed—by probiotics.

How did I do it? Glad you asked. I make my own probiotic drink by soaking nuts and seeds and drinking the soak water and by using the pulp from juicing to make a sauerkraut drink. Fermented foods are known to be much more effective at building healthy bacteria than taking probiotic supplements.

My favorite has to be beet and red cabbage. All you do is fill a gallon glass jar about a third of the way up with your favorite pulp, add water and wait for it to "make." It is temperature sensitive, meaning it makes much more quickly in a warm environment than a cool one. When it expands, it's ready. You can also taste or smell it to see if it is ready. This is a "wild" culture, no need to "seed" it—it just grows when the right conditions are met. You may also see that it is ready by noticing a bit of mold or bubbles on the top. Just spoon off the mold and strain as normal.

To prepare the drink for consumption, you just strain off the liquid from the vegetable pulp. I use a course strainer, pressing the pulp against the strainer with a large spoon. I then progress to a fine strainer. I put the liquid in a sealed glass container. It keeps for weeks, possibly even months refrigerated.

Most cultures throughout the world have some kind of take on sauerkraut, which is a German word for the cabbage or other vegetable culture. The Japanese have "kimchee" also made from cabbage, the Inuit bury seal flipper in the permafrost for a year or so, and enjoy their probiotic "stinkflipper". Maybe that's why it's called culture!

Anyway, it's nice to have some use for the juicing pulp, other than compost. I've tried lots of different veggies. The ones with a high sugar content will make the fastest. Japanese sweet potato makes a good one. Carrot seems to be too sugary. It gets thick, and can expand so fast it overflows its jar and makes a mess if you're not careful. No juicer? No problem. Just use a blender or a food processor and grind up any veggie that strikes your fancy. Experiment with different vegetables.

I will go over the process step by step in the back of the book. I will also take you through the nut and seed making process. They are both very simple, but I've noticed that folks like to have a step-by-step description. I'm all about showing you how easy all this really is.

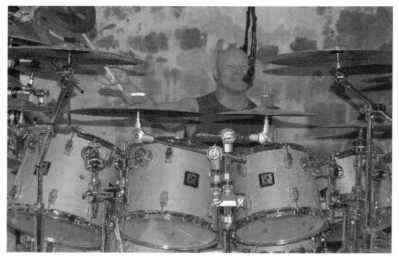

"Music...next to silence that which comes closest to expressing the inexpressible."

\- John McLaughlin

"The more I see, the less I know for sure."

\- John Lennon

CHAPTER 11
FOOD COMBINING

N ow, we need to talk about a major component of building (or destroying) health that is seldom talked about and little appreciated. It is as obscure a subject as probiotics were a decade ago. In time, it will surely be accepted as important as probiotics, which has gone mainstream faster than anything in the health field in my memory.

I'm talking about food combining. This is not a new topic. I first read about the importance of not giving your body so many complex combinations of foods to digest at one time in the 70s. Let's go back to basic anatomy/evolution to explain this concept. Through all of human evolution, until recent times, no human ate every day. The body became very adept at storing any extra calories as fat for leaner times. The body also became very efficient at extracting all the nutrients it so desperately needed from the little food received. The body had to survive scarcity far more often than not.

One thing it did not have to deal with, and so, has no adaptation to, are combinations of different foods in one meal. This may well be a new concept to you because when we think of combining foods, we think only of how they taste together. Sad to say, some, if not most of our cherished food concoctions, are the hardest to digest, if they are digested at all. Consider this: as hunter-gatherers, we almost never ate foods in combination. If we dug roots, we had roots. If we found berries, we had berries, if we killed an animal, we had meat. Man has been eating meat for thousands of years, but that does not mean it's our natural food. To even have a prayer of digesting it, we must cook, or otherwise treat it. We are also much more susceptible to parasites in the meat than omnivores. Ever heard of an omnivore with trichinosis or tularemia? Back to combining.

Our bodies evolved a complex system to digest the different foods we consume. Here's how it works. First, we must chew food well, which already presents problems because to modern man chewing has become a lost art form. People ask me if, being on a liquid diet, I miss chewing. I usually say, "Don't you?" I tell them I get all of the enjoyment of eating with none of the work. We've all been told that we need to chew more/better, but few of us do a very good job. We may assume that if we don't chew enough that somehow the stomach will do it. It won't. If you don't chew well enough with your teeth, the job will not be done.

So now, we come to the second stop in the digestive process, the stomach. Most people think digestion occurs in the stomach. Actually, it's a holding chamber, where some general "softening up" acids like hydrochloric and pepsin start digestion. The food is all mixed up in a mash of different ingredients. If you drank with this meal though, even this pre-digestion cannot occur. The fluid you drank has diluted these acids and enzymes. The liquid must first be shuttled out of the stomach before anything can happen to the food. This slows digestion down, keeping you feeling full longer, but as you'll see, slowing digestion is not what we want.

So now, after the liquid moves along on its way through the small intestine to the colon, leaving the food, pre-digestion can start in the stomach. Then, the real digestion happens in the small intestine, particularly the middle part, called the jejunum. The part of the small intestine the stomach empties into is called the duodenum; it is a very interesting place, housing some 70% - 80% of your immune system. It has Peyers

Patches, which are raised nodules, kind of like birdhouses for probiotics, giving them a place to grow and proliferate. These probiotics, along with white blood cells and a few other players ARE your immune system.[1]

The last stage that feeds into the colon is the ilium. Here's the punchline, every different type of food requires a different enzymatic and chemical action. In other words, an enzyme called amylase digests starch, Protein by lipase. So food, even though it mixes in the stomach, is taken in turn by the small intestine. Fruit is always the first, because it is the easiest to digest, then vegetables. Starch, which takes quite a long time to digest is next. Protein, being the hardest to break down, is last, and it ain't getting any fresher.

This is why we have so much indigestion and heartburn. It's not your heart that's burning; it's your gut.[2] This also explains why eating a large "mixed" meal makes you so tired; you are using a lot of energy to process all this complexity. Remember, your body has no evolutionary adaptation to this mishmash of food. Many different metabolic waste products are formed when food hangs around in this warm moist environment. The longer the food hangs out, the more pathogens can feed and grow on it, and the more waste products are produced.

Never before modern times have we had the variety of food at one meal, except for kings perhaps. They were never known for their healthy states or their sweet dispositions either.

Turns out that some of the most common food combinations are the worst. Protein and starch is the absolute worst. Worse still are all of the food groups together, like a sandwich with lettuce and tomato, or a pizza. You have no doubt trained your body to deal with this abuse on a daily basis. The bad news is that oftentimes, maybe most of the time, the protein is not digested at all, going straight through to the colon and sometimes staying there, why? You ate again before digestion was complete. Your body had no choice but to send it down the line.[3]

We have been conditioned to eat three times a day. You get hungry long before the stomach is empty. It you eat simple meals, without drinking with them, this will not be a problem. This is another reason why fasting, even for a day or two, is so beneficial. I read that George Burns, who lived to be 100, despite his martinis and cigars, fasted one day every week, as well as eating very little by American standards. Fasting gives the body a rest and time to clean up.

Often times when you're hungry, you're actually feeling the symptoms of detoxing start. You may feel weak, irritable, or tired. This is been referred to as "toxic hunger".[4] Many of us have never felt real hunger in our lives, we have just gotten used to eating when we feel a little hungry or a little lethargic. If you're trying to eat less or fast and you feel hungry, try drinking a substantial amount of liquid. Many times when you feel hungry you are really thirsty. Most people go through life in a state of partial dehydration. A great experiment to do on yourself is to drink when you feel hungry and see what happens. It is very easy to skip meals this way. While we want to eat as much as we can of the healthy foods, skipping meals, you will find, is a great way to fine tune your metabolism and increase your energy level.

Here's the way to revitalize your digestive system to keep metabolic waste and slow digestion from aging you. Eat simply. Be well hydrated before you eat and don't drink for 3 or so hours after eating. The more complex the meal, the longer you need to wait. If you drink before the meal is completely digested, digestion will slow or stop until the liquid is sent on its way to the colon. We are creatures of habit. The trick is to pick the habits you want and cultivate those.

The good habits are much easier to cultivate than the bad ones. Why? Because they are what your body wants. It will work with you if you just give it some breathing room. You have given it no choice but to make the best of what you throw at it. What a miraculous instrument it is to be able to do that! As you get cleaner and healthier, you will find yourself wondering how other people and even your former self can carry on that way. Actually, your former life becomes like a forgotten dream; you won't be able to recall how you used to feel. At least that was my experience. Even though I started young, I did grow up on cereal for breakfast and school lunches, not to mention fast food. Again, the difference between eating some and none is dramatic. Likewise, the difference between eating easy to digest combinations and giving your body a bunch of mishmash is profound—and a lot more fun. You will be rewarded greatly, I promise.

Your body will begin to wake up and talk to you. Let's say you stopped drinking with or shortly after meals for a while, then slipped up and drank too soon after or with a meal. You will feel fullness and discomfort as you never did before. You feel it now because you gave the body a taste of what it's like not to drink with meals. Now, the body is talking. If you listen to your body, great things will follow. You will continue to be guided to greater and greater health and well-being. You will feel so much calm and peace, while having virtually unlimited energy, words cannot describe. Guess I'd better try 'cause you bought this book. All I can do is share my experience.

As a young dude, I was reading everything I could get my hands on about health and diet. I had noticed such a dramatic difference in the way I felt in giving up first meat and fish then dairy, and finally flour products, that I was excited to know more and more. I read about food combining and immediately put it into practice. It made so much sense to me that we never evolved with complicated combinations. A book I read also suggested what it called the "no breakfast plan", whereby you don't eat in the morning, instead extending the nightly fast into the day. It suggested if you were used to eating a meal in the morning, just eat some fruit instead. I was always a big breakfast kinda guy, but it took only a few days for my body to adapt and to reward me beyond my wildest dreams. I had so much energy; I couldn't believe it.

I have been listening to my body ever since. That's how the liquid diet happened. It's where my body wants to be. The rewards are beyond description. I don't recommend this to anyone, as I've said. To me, the ultimate diet is raw food only, but you don't have to go raw to age in reverse. You will naturally gravitate to eating more and more raw food as you get cleaner and your taste develops for what your body wants. Not eating salt will help to revitalize your sense of taste. Rawsome.

I used to go to raw food meet up groups to give my card out and offer advice and support to those who were drawn to eating raw. These were potlucks and everyone brought a dish to share. Some of the concoctions were very elaborate indeed. I heard more than one person complain of a full, almost indigested feeling from eating all that complexity. You could tell the ones who had been raw or nearly raw for a long time by the few different things on their plates.

The most natural way to eat of all is to eat one thing at a time. The so called a mono-food diet. A guy at one of these meetings did a talk about the benefit of what he called sequential eating, whereby you eat different foods in order one at a time even though it gets mixed up in the stomach. I guess he thought digestion was almost instantaneous.

As you get into this, you will see how fast change occurs when you work with your body. Ideally, and I experienced this, you can go from plate to toilet in four or so hours, leaving food no time to ferment and putrefy.

Ever wonder why that food smells so good going in and so bad coming out? What happens to it in your body to make it smell so bad? Remember, certain non-foods will always smell bed coming out. Meat will always be dead decaying flesh. No matter how clean you get, it will always smell bad coming out. I had that experience when I tried wild caught salmon years ago. Ever the experimenter, I had read about how great it was for you with all the right essential fatty acids and red pigment from wonderful marine algae called astaxanthin[5] which has all kinds of benefits. I'm not tied idealistically to being a vegan, so I gave it a try. OMG, it made my poop stink! Dead fish is so stinky. No more of that.

So, let's explore some more the question of why does the freshest most delectable vegetable matter smell so good going in and so bad coming out of your body? Most people have never pondered this. It is a profound question though, one that will shed much light on the process of aging and decline. When most people think of the worst possible stench imaginable, they would think of human waste. It will no doubt surprise you to learn, if you can believe it, that some of us have "shit that don't stink"! Again, I will ask you not to believe me, but to experience.

So, what is it that stinks so badly? Well, if you eat dead things, you'll smell like death. In addition, it's due to bacteria that find a perfect breeding ground in all that warm, moist fermenting matter hanging around much longer than is healthy. When you make it complicated for your digestive system, bad things happen. Or should I say bad smells happen. They come out all kinds of ways. What do you think bad breath is all about? Body odor? When you're clean, you don't need deodorant. I've had folks tell me I smelled like coconut or celery. A lot of the stuff people eat is literally rotting inside them. Don't let this happen to you —anymore. You hopefully, don't know this is happening now; I didn't either until I felt the difference. Simplify things for your body and great things will happen. Speed up digestion and feel the difference.

Speeding up digestion has another olfactory benefit, less gas. What kind of gas specifically? Methane. The reason one cow puts out more greenhouse gas in a year than an SUV is that methane is up to 50 times more damaging to the ozone layer than CO2.[6] Do your part to slow global warming...emit less methane. Actually, I should say, produce less. When it's in there, you want to let it out. Do not let it absorb into your body. As Ben Franklin said, "Fart proudly."

A method I developed and have now perfected is loudly clear your throat when you let fly in polite company. Just takes practice. Do whatever you have to; let it out. This gas is emitted by decaying matter. Still don't believe you have stuff hanging out in there? What we call heartburn is methane produced in the stomach from all the stuff that is hanging out there and not getting any fresher. Belching likewise can be methane escaping caused by the same thing. It can also be showing you that your probiotic supplement is working.

This leads me to talk about a substance that has gotten much press in the last few decades - Fiber. How many hideous breakfast cereals claim to be 'heart healthy' because they contain fiber. Too many to count. Actually, there has never been a study linking fiber in and of itself to heart health....or any other kind of health for that matter.[7]

One way fiber is said to be of benefit is by slowing down digestion. Fiber allows a more gradual absorption of sugars from food, thereby not spiking the blood sugar and causing an inflammatory chain reaction. We must do something to keep blood sugar surges from occurring, but slowing down digestion is not the answer. We want food to move through quickly, so fermentation and putrefaction don't occur. Also, we want food to digest before we eat something else and push the partially undigested meal down the line before it's fully digested. Remember this is a warm, moist environment we're talking about. Getting back to the fiber rap, studies that suggest fiber is beneficial usually take the form of pitting a non-fibrous food or group of foods against more fibrous foods.

The fibrous food is by nature healthier and thus shows positive results. No animal food has fiber. If you eat many salads, beans, fruit, veggies, nuts and seeds, you will have all the fiber you need. People ask me sometimes "If you're on a liquid diet where do you get your fiber?" That's kind of the point. My body doesn't want fiber. I don't advocate this diet for anyone else. Please indulge in all the healthy fiber you want. Don't worry that you're not getting enough. No need to supplement it. Just eat your veggies.

A lot of what we think of as fiber is just more goo going into your body. Vegetables that are cooked more than just a light steaming or sautéing have had their beneficial fiber turned into a paste. Oat bran and the like is just more sticky stuff. If you eat a healthy diet with lots of vegetables that are not overcooked, you will have all the fiber you need. Not that you really need any, but you probably think you do, and that's okay. Trying to get more fiber into your diet in the hopes of moving food through your digestive system, especially your colon, more efficiently is like swallowing a spider to catch a fly. Putting more volume in to get volume out, doesn't make any sense. Liquid intake is the real fix to this problem. All you have to do, in my opinion, is just eat your vegetables and don't overcook them.

So many of the doctors I have referred to in this book state that fiber is very important in the diet, but that you should get your fiber from food not from fiber supplements. In my own body, I have found that fiber is not something it wants. That's why the liquid diet happened; for me fiber has no value whatsoever. Everybody says that fiber is so important. This has not been my experience, but who am I to argue with everybody? My advice? Eat lots of fiber in the form of vegetables.

The concept of fiber was originally brought to modern consciousness by one person. He was a missionary in Africa, who noticed the native population had zero cancer of any kind with little or no heart disease.[8] He reasoned it was because their diets were full of what he called roughage. It makes sense, but the evidence is just not there that fiber is the reason for their good health.

These people were living in small communities, close to their neighbors and friends with lifetime relationships and very little turmoil other than being what we would call poor. Actually, the people who live the longest are usually the poorest. Calorie restriction or CR, as its become known, has been shown to increase lifespan in any species it is tested on by 50% or more. We may see them as poor, but living close to the land, working hard, and enjoying close relationships, while eating very simply and sparsely, looks to me like an awesome way to live. I wouldn't know. It's probably a lot harder life than it looks. But healthy? Oh yeah.

I have found that food combining does not matter nearly as much if you consume your food in liquid form. I like to make nut milk and then add frozen fruit to it to make a wonderful milkshake. A recipe I have turned many people on to, is what I call cashew ice cream. All you do is make cashew milk very thick, like a pudding consistency, and add frozen cherries to it.

The recipe for cashew milk is in the appendix. You can use any fruit you like. Cashews are such a wonderful nut to experiment with because they are so sweet and tasty and require no prep like soaking. Cashews are also high in the amino acid tryptophan.[9] Which has a calming effect on the body. It has long been used as a sleep aid. We can all use some more calmness in our lives.

As we clean up our diets, getting rid of the foods that were aging us, we naturally make room for the foods that will age us in reverse. Green leafy vegetables are number one here. Be sure to eat a huge salad every day. I recommend making the salad the main course. The downside of eating a lot of salad is it requires a lot of chewing. Your jaws may get tired. While this is good exercise for the facial muscles, there is an easier way. Put your salad through a food processor. Food that is not well chewed will not be well absorbed. The food processor works great in this capacity because you get to enjoy the taste of the food without working so hard. The added benefit is better and faster digestion. Or, you can make a lettuce soup by blending lettuce on high by adding some form of liquid to taste plus spices or other favorite ingredients then warming on the stove.

When we are eating the healthy foods—the age reversal foods, we can eat as much as we want. Try to keep it simple for the body by not eating too much variety at a meal, but there's no need to stress too much about this. Soon your body will lead you in the direction it wants to go. The more you listen to its voice, the louder it will get. We have in effect silenced its voice by eating what our addictions dictated to us. As we give the body more and more breathing room, it wakes up and starts to talk to us. Our free will can always override what the body is asking for. Great things happen when we listen to and honor what the body wants. Just be sure it's not your addictions talking.

I have heard people say that since they were craving a certain food, it meant the body needed that type of food. Probably not. It was more likely their addictions in one of addiction's many disguises talking. As you get cleaner and more in tune with your body you will be able to trust more and more that it is the body and not your addiction talking to you.

Remember that the so-called "hunger headache", and the irritability and lack of energy you may feel from not eating for a while, is showing you how toxic your body actually is. These symptoms often appear even when the stomach is not even empty. Dr. Fuhrman calls this phenomenon "toxic hunger". As we continue to cleanse, the body continues to wake up and guide us more and more surely. We will be able to eat less because we won't be eating to keep these symptoms away.

Keep in mind that it is very beneficial to skip meals. Remember eating every day is a modern phenomenon. It is much more natural to miss meals and take days where you only consume liquid. Most people in developed countries have never known true hunger. You may feel weak, irritable, or tired when you haven't eaten for a while. This is due to detoxification. Your body always endeavors to clean itself of toxins when you give it some space by not eating. When you give it a break from digesting it starts cleansing. As you get cleaner, you will come to enjoy the feeling of being light, not weighed down by a full stomach. Missing meals is a huge step in the direction of age reversal.

If you are consciously trying to eat less by skipping meals, and you feel hungry, try involving yourself in something that takes your mind off your temporary hunger. You will find that all of a sudden you don't feel hungry anymore. You start to get in touch with your body and your ability to influence it and its ability to influence you.

I had an experience soon after I adopted the liquid diet. I was with my family at Christmas. While we were at the table and everyone except me was eating the Christmas feast, I felt a faint pang of hunger. I thought to myself "OMG I love this feeling of lightness!" Most people equate that feeling of emptiness with depravity. I have had people ask me if my liquid diet "fills me up?" I have come to very much enjoy a lighter way of being. Back when I ate one raw meal a day, I used to enjoy eating until I was full. I have found that once I got away from that feeling of fullness, and got used to a lighter state, I never wanted to be "full" again.

One more thought. "Chewing" liquid food, like juice or not milks is very beneficial. Swishing a mouthful around or, as I like to say, chewing it, infuses it with saliva, facilitating better digestion. Drinking slowly, as well as eating slowly is very beneficial. Endeavor to develop the habit of drinking well before eating, and just as importantly—drinking a large amount at a time, like a meal. This applies to water as well. If you drink a large amount, peristalsis is stimulated. If you get in the habit of drinking a large amount of liquid and then sit on the toilet, great things will happen. There is been a lot of press about how we need to drink more water.

You see so many people now carrying bottles with them and sipping throughout the day. While this is better than being dehydrated, the real magic happens when you drink large amounts at a time. I drink half-gallon at a time virtually every time I drink. (I almost never drink just water because my meals are all liquid) Try to drink at least a quart every time you drink something... and drink it on an empty stomach, well before eating a meal. See what happens.

When you are well hydrated by drinking a large amount at a time, you will not be tempted to drink too soon after a meal. One of the greatest health habits to cultivate is to drink a large amount at a time every time you drink. When you are in the habit of drinking large amounts at a time you will not be able to drink before digestion of the last meal is complete, as it will make you too full.

We want our food digested quickly and completely. That way there is no time for it to ferment and for toxins to form. If you drink with meals or too soon after (before digestion is complete), your digestion is much slower and not as complete.

You will not be able to drink the large amount I am suggesting if the stomach is not empty. This is why most people sip throughout the day—their stomachs are almost never empty. Digestion is a very long process because they slow it down by drinking with and too soon after meals. Drinking large amounts of water is very detoxifying. Water is the solvent and the medium for nearly all of the body's (and the Earth's) processes. Get in the habit of drinking like a camel—a lot at a time. This is especially great for athletes.

A little story: last year I was about to do an all day hike in the Arizona desert. I didn't want to carry liquid, as I wanted to feel light and free, and not to have to carry anything. To prepare for the day's exertions, I drank a half gallon of juice, followed by a trip to the toilet; a short time later, I repeated this. So now, I'm tanked up and evacuated. I went all day without drinking. I used to do long distance trail runs (before I got the titanium rod in my leg) where I used the same strategy. I have trained my body to take large amounts of liquid and use it throughout the day. These bodies are ours to nurture and to train in any way we want. What will you train yours to do?

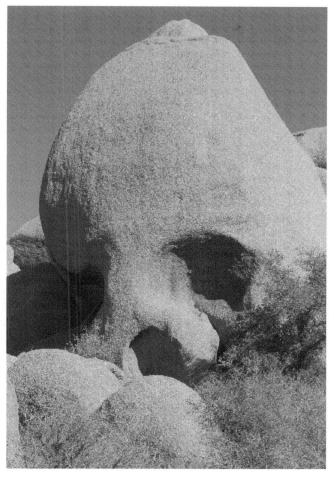

Skull Rock, Joshua Tree National Monument

"To live is the rarest thing in the world. Most people exist, that is all."

\- Oscar Wilde

CHAPTER 12
ATHEROSCLEROSIS

M ost of us are born with a perfectly healthy, flawlessly intact endothelium. The endothelium is a one cell thick layer that lines all of our arteries and blood vessels. Arteries carry blood away from the heart to be circulated throughout the body. Veins return the blood to the heart to be re-oxygenated. When you are born your circulatory system is free of obstruction and your endothelium is clean and functioning perfectly. Arteries and veins are not just pipes that blood flows through, but dynamic organs. They are even more profoundly affected by our poor food choices than most other organ systems.

As we age the endothelium, once perfectly smooth and clean, becomes clogged or in medical terminology, occluded. When we talk about occlusion in the circulatory system, we are talking about the endothelium, as it is the lining. The occlusions are sticking to the surface of the endothelium. As I discussed in the chapter on dairy, the wrong kind of calcium causes bone growth (ossification) on the endothelium within the artery.[1] The primary cause of occluded arteries is the wrong kind of dietary fat. As you probably know, there are two main types of cholesterol: HDL and LDL. The letters stand for high density lipoprotein and low density lipoprotein. What this means is that the low-density variety is small particles of cholesterol which clump together easily, causing occlusion, thus it is termed bad cholesterol.

HDL actually removes arterial clogging. If we increase our HDL and lower our LDL, we can clean our circulatory system up. This is a further example of how regeneration (age reversal) happens.[2] Cellular waste products are released into the bloodstream for filtration and excretion through the kidneys. Toxicity is an often-overlooked cause of endothelial aging. The less toxins we carry and circulate the less arterial aging occurs. Also damaging to the endothelium and therefore the artery are elevated glucose from too much sugar, especially the kind we get from flour products. All that circulating insulin, which is not picked up because the receptors are partially or fully shut down as discussed in our chapter on wheat, is damaging to the endothelium as well. Triglycerides are a factor, and are not only created by the wrong kind of fat. The wrong kind of carbohydrate elevates them also.[3]

Homocysteine and C-reactive protein are two inflammatory markers that more enlightened doctors look for along with high LDL cholesterol as risk factors for heart disease.[4] It is now being appreciated that inflammation is a major player in all disease systems especially those of the circulatory system. Many doctors, probably most, are still fixated on the cholesterol number. In any case, the real cure is the same. If you want to get rid of the main cause of arterial aging, get rid of the substances that cause occlusion, Animal fats.

Trans fats are probably even worse. Most of us have heard by now how bad these fats are. They're still widely used in prepared foods such as salad dressing and virtually any potato chip, cookie, or cracker. New York City, I understand, has outlawed the use of all trans fats in restaurants. Almost all brands of commercial oils contain trans fats. Animal fats, as bad as they are, still occur in nature. Trans fats are manufactured.[5] Most people savvy enough to be reading a book on age reversal know about trans fats. If you haven't heard yet, I suggest you learn more. The main caution I would like to offer is not to substitute margarine for butter. Back in the 70s, margarine was touted as a health food. It is virtually nothing but trans-fat. This is another example of how we must educate ourselves. Or else.

Life Extension Foundation magazine, by no means a vegetarian publication, has this to say about the inflammatory marker (indicator of inflammation in the body) homocysteine: "High homocysteine is associated with increasing age, consumption of animal protein, smoking, postmenopausal state, sedentary lifestyle, decreased kidney function, deficiencies of B vitamins, or with certain genetic abnormalities." Once again, animal protein is at the heart of this particular attack on your heart. We can absolutely control this variable. High homocysteine is right up there with cholesterol as a causative factor in arterial occlusion and the resultant heart disease.

Low testosterone is emerging from the research as a factor in endothelial aging/clogging. Low testosterone is associated with loss of insulin sensitivity, loss of muscle mass, increased abdominal fat, decreased libido, arteriosclerosis, and increased incidence of cardiovascular disease. The body's manufacture of this hormone, like many other beneficial hormones and cofactors, goes way down as we age. Most people do not have enough, especially men. Just having excess visceral (belly) fat decreases free testosterone.

Testosterone creams are prescribed to many men and some women. The problem with supplementing a hormone or neurotransmitter directly is that the body slows down or even stops producing it. Better to give the body the raw materials to make its own testosterone. These include ginger, maca, zinc, and selenium. Soy, which contains a phytoestrogen, wipes out free testosterone.[6] 'Free' meaning circulating and able to be used, as opposed to the bound form of testosterone.

A quick note to middle-aged women in the dating pool: if a guy you meet has more than just a little belly fat, chances are he's impotent, at least some of the time. Belly fat is one characteristic that determines one's biological age. Another is the amount of occlusion that has occurred in the arteries, and the speed at which it is progressing.

The arteries are under constant attack on many fronts. Not only high cholesterol, but also high homocysteine, as well as at least 18 other major health players, enumerated below, are occluding your arteries and eating away at your quality of life.

All these factors help explain why most people who undergo coronary bypass to replace an occluded artery, or receive a stent or any other invasive heart surgery, often need another one within five or so years. If you don't address the lifestyle choices that create the blockage, the arteries will again become occluded. Duh. Most doctors don't do much in the way of counseling people on the lifestyle changes that keep occlusion from happening. They just do the surgery and send the person on their way. Since most people look to doctors for health information, they are very poorly served indeed. A return trip to the surgeon's table is all but guaranteed.

HDL, the "good" cholesterol can actually clean out your arteries. An enzyme called PON-1 is attached to its surface. As we age, levels of PON-1 markedly decline thereby reducing the ability of HDL to protect against heart attack and stroke. This helps explain why the rate of occlusion tends to speed up dramatically as people age. Lipid peroxidation is a free radical reaction that severely damages cell membranes and causes many degenerative diseases. PON-1 blocks this destructive cascade of events.[7]

Two saviors have emerged to activate PON-1 and save us from the ravages of LDL cholesterol and its attendant occlusion of our arteries. Pomegranate and tart cherry juice.

You can get either one in extract form as a supplement or you can just drink the juice. Pomegranate extracts have been shown to promote cholesterol outflow, to enhance natural antioxidant systems, and to protect us from oxidant damage and inflammation.[8]

Here's a quote from the latest issue of Life Extension Magazine: "Inflammatory molecules contribute to the onset of diabetes, arthritis, obesity, heart disease, Alzheimer's, and cancer—virtually every degenerative disease. Tart cherries protect the liver and offer unrivaled direct inflammamomodulatory (modifies inflammation) effect. In fact, some scientists have stated tart cherries have the highest antioxidant and anti-inflammatory content of any food. They also increase the activity of your body's key antioxidant enzyme superoxide dismutase (SOD). Tart cherries have a high anthocyanin content. The real secret to their effectiveness against many inflammatory diseases is their broad range of anthocyanins. As a result, tart cherries synergistically target a remarkably wide spectrum of oxidation and inflammation induced diseases. Tart cherries allow aging individuals to block an extremely wide range of degenerative diseases—at their oxidative inflammatory root!" Life Extension Foundation carries a tart cherry extract supplement I have been taking because tart cherry also helps with muscle soreness and recovery after intense exercise. Check them out at www.lef.org.

One of the main hallmarks of aging is artery occlusion. The state of occlusion in the arteries is used as a direct measurement of your biological age.[9] In most people, this occluding process goes on without interruption at a steady rate. In most people, this process does not reverse itself. Science now knows how it can. We must lower our LDL number to somewhere close to 100. We must raise our HDL and take these plant helpers to assist it in achieving cholesterol outflow.

You see? Age reversal IS possible. Most people will never do this. They will continue to eat the substances they are addicted to. They will never get to take the journey that you are about to take. Don't let your addictions prevent you from accessing these miracles. Actually, there's nothing miraculous about it. Once we start to work with our bodies instead of against them, so-called miracles are inevitable and certain.

I couldn't close this chapter without telling you about one more substance that can help save us from the fate of clogged arteries. It's also being used to prevent and cure arthritis, colitis, Crohn's disease, and brain degeneration of all kinds. It mentioned in the Bible as frankincense. We know it as Boswellia.

Boswellia has long been used for arthritis relief. It has lately been becoming known as a general and very powerful anti-inflammatory. It is getting attention also as a cancer fighter. It actually shuts down the master inflammation regulatory complex NF-kappaB in tumors. Boswellia can cause cell death (apoptosis) to cancer cells, putting cancer into remission.[10] We are seeing again how inflammation is at the heart of virtually all disease systems.

Atherosclerosis, since it narrows blood vessels and occludes arteries, is a major player in cognitive decline. Decreasing blood flow to the brain certainly cannot be a good thing. Stroke occurs when blood flow to the brain decreases enough to cause permanent damage. Since inflammation is a component in the buildup of plaque, anything that helps to quell the fires of inflammation in the body is going to keep your arteries from hardening as well. A quote from an article in Life Extension Magazine: "Boswellia extracts are beginning to show promise in preventing the inflammation that contributes to atherosclerosis. In rats fed a high-fat and atherosclerosis promoting diet, supplementation with Boswellia extract significantly lowered total cholesterol by up to 48%, and increased beneficial HDL cholesterol by up to 30%. In the same study, liver and kidney functions return to near-normal levels."

To further quote the life extension article: "Chronic inflammation also induces changes in the function of platelets, the tiny cell fragments responsible for initiating blood clotting. Inflammatory signals trigger platelets to become increasingly sticky, causing them to adhere to vessel walls and eventually blocking blood flow to produce a heart attack or stroke. Boswellia extracts have now been shown to significantly inhibit platelet activation and subsequent clumping."

Boswellia has even been shown to regenerate arthritic joints. Of the most interest to our aging population may be its ability to regenerate our brains. Check out this quote: "A component of Boswella, a resin called incensoleacetate, inhibits NF-kappaB, and has been shown to inhibit the gene expression of inflammatory mediators in an animal model of traumatic brain injury. This effect also inhibits degenerative changes in the hippocampus, one of the brains chief memory processing areas. Boswellic acids have also been found to stimulate hippocampal cells to grow new highly branching projections called neuritis. Neurites are projections that brain cells use to contact multiple other cells to advance cognition and memory. This important study is disapproving the outdated belief that brain tissue cannot regenerate and gives a ray of hope to those currently suffering from degenerative brain disorders that are believed to be incurable." That's what I'm talkin' about——age reversal.

There is no reason to let our arteries fill with plaque and our brains fill with fog. We have the tools now in the form of these plant helpers, and the knowledge to regenerate areas of our bodies previously considered beyond our ability to influence. New research keeps showing that age reversal is not only possible but also inevitable if we will just start to work with the body instead of against it. Our world is filled with toxins our grandparents and even our parents never had to deal with. Even so, we can be healthier than any generation that has ever gone before us. We have many more dietary supplements and much more knowledge than any generation has had.

Some of this new knowledge has to do with inflammation. As I have said before, many doctors are not on board with this yet. Too many are still focused mostly on cholesterol as a risk factor for heart disease. The research is showing inflammation is a factor in cancer as well. Inflammation is part of the body's immune response. Somehow, the immune system, through inflammation, attacks the body. How does this happen? Why does this happen? Why does it seem to be happening so much more than it used to? We never used to hear the term "autoimmune disease". This is a medical mystery. It is starting to be unraveled though. It looks like anything that irritates the body, like the isoflavone in soy that activates histamines, causes an inflammatory response.[11]

A very interesting experiment was done several decades ago by a researcher named Frances Pottenger.[12] He fed cats raw meat, and then measured their white blood cell count. It was not elevated in the cats fed raw meat. When he fed the cats cooked meat the white cell count went way up. White blood cells are also called macrophages. They hunt down and kill invading pathogens. The fact that they were elevated after a cooked meal points to cooked food being perceived by the body as a threat. I don't know of any research that has continued along this line. Surely, it would be very illuminating if more work were done in this direction.

I recently did some research on Crohn's disease and colitis.[13] These seem to be on the rise these days. What happens in many cases of Crohn's is that the intestine in one or more areas is eaten away by the immune system. Why? It must be that the body perceives some sort of threat and is activating an immune response. To what? It's a very interesting question. I don't claim to have the answer. But it seems obvious that our unnatural diets, full of their caustic irritants and anti-nutrients are causing the immune system to react. All I know for sure is that "miracles" happen you get rid of these irritants.

In an age when most doctors are still fixated on cholesterol as the be-all indicator of heart disease risk, 18 separate risk factors have been identified. I would like to briefly share these with you.

1. Low EPA/DHA: These essential fatty acids that are synthesized by the body when it is given sufficient omega-3, 7, and 9 fatty acids. EPA/DHA is the reason fish oil is considered so healthy. Some health writers will tell you that you can only get these from fish oil. Others say the body synthesizes EPA/DHA from omega-3 fatty acid. EPA/DHA are essential for proper brain function. Certainly, deficiency in them is a risk factor for cognitive decline. I do not myself consume fish oil, as I feel it is too full of toxins to be healthy, even though I have read that the toxins tend to stay in the meat, and do not readily bind to the oil. If it were true that the only source of EPA/DHA were fish oil, and that the body could not synthesize it. I would not have any, and would not have proper brain function. After you finish this book, you can form your own opinion about whether I have proper brain function or not.

2. Elevated C-reactive protein: This may be the new gold standard instead of elevated LDL cholesterol.[14] It is

used as an inflammatory marker, showing how much inflammation is present in the body. Inflammation, we now know as a causative risk factor in virtually every disease system.

3. Excess LDL: The wrong fats clog your arteries. The letters LDL stands for low-density lipoprotein. This means that the particles of cholesterol are small and easily adhere to the vascular system. Not only your arteries but also the heart itself is affected. More enlightened heart specialists suggest that the LDL numbers considered normal by mainstream medicine are too high. They recommend we keep it below 100.

4. Excess insulin: When we spike our blood sugar by consuming sugar in any form, especially wheat, insulin pours into the blood stream by the pancreas to put out this inflammatory fire. Circulating insulin in the high amounts necessary to stop this inflammatory cascade cause many problems in the body. Even fruit juice can cause this blood sugar surge. The take-home message is; eat foods low on the glycemic index.

5. Low HDL: The "good cholesterol—high-density lipoprotein can actually clear the arteries of the damage that LDL does. Plant foods do not contain, or cause the body to produce LDL. It should come as no surprise that plant foods are high in the good cholesterol. Bottom line: eat low on the food chain.

6. High glucose: We eat way too much sugar. Too much sugar of course causes obesity, but that is just the beginning of the problems sugar causes. Check out the documentary "Fed Up". It terms sugar "the new tobacco". However, as we now know table sugar is not the only problem. Flour products are actually worse.

7. Nitric oxide deficit: I'll quote from Life Extension Magazine:" As humans age, endothelial function becomes altered. Due to a variety of insults, depletion of nitric oxide occurs in the endothelium. One consequence of nitric oxide depletion is the inability of the arteries to expand and contract with youthful elasticity. The continual stiffening and occlusion of aged arteries is the number one health risk that people in Western societies face. In order to maintain healthy arteriole dilation, the endothelium has to manufacture enough nitric oxide. Impairment in nitric oxide release by the aging endothelium causes arterial dysfunction." Pomegranate extract or juice will assist the endothelium in making this vital component.

8. Insufficient vitamin D: Vitamin D has been likened to a hormone that your body cannot produce, carrying out many functions throughout the body. We will cover vitamin D in more detail later. Suffice to say now that most people are severely deficient in vitamin D; and it is one of the cheapest supplements you can buy, The D3 form is the one you want. It is absolute rubbish that you can get all you need from the sun, especially if your skin is dark, or like most of us you don't get outside in the sun much anyway. So much for the idea that the sun is bad for us. You could probably more accurately say that lack of sunlight causes cancer, and heart disease.[15]

9. Low vitamin K: Here's a nutrient that like vitamin D, doesn't occur in many foods. Vitamin D you almost certainly need to supplement. Vitamin K you will be getting in abundance if you eat green leafy vegetables. I'm hoping that as you get rid of the animal products and wheat from your diet, you will start eating a lot more salads and vegetables. These super foods protect

your arteries and the rest of your body from oxidative, viral, and every other kind of attack. Vitamin K especially protects from ossification in your arteries, by too much of the wrong kind of calcium. The blessing that vitamin K brings to your arteries endothelium cannot be overstated.[16]

10. Excess estrogen: Phytoestrogen as found in soy food certainly must be avoided. Excess estrogen can wipe out your circulating or "free" testosterone. Not that this is the only problem with excess estrogen. One reason for soy's reputation as a health food is that phytoestrogen is perceived as a good thing for older women who are low in estrogen. More enlightened doctors these days are not just prescribing supplementation of hormones like estrogen. They are testing actual levels of certain hormones and only supplementing the ones you are actually deficient in. The "shotgun approach" to hormone replacement is falling by the wayside. Thank God. It's not enough for supplemental hormones to be "Bio-identical"; they have to be given in doses that address actual need. Or even better, optimize your diet, and watch hormone levels normalize themselves.

11. Excess triglycerides: Like cholesterol, the body manufactures triglycerides. Most people have levels of triglycerides that are excessively high due to consumption of the wrong kind of fat. Interesting new research has shown that excess sugar in all its forms can raise triglyceride levels as well. It seems no matter what risk factor we are talking about, animal products and wheat are the primary causes. Consumption of vegetables and fruits, with large amounts of nuts, seeds, beans, mushrooms, seaweed, and onions reverse it.

12. Low free testosterone: It is now known that low testosterone predisposes you to heart disease. It was thought until recently that high testosterone predisposed you to prostate cancer. That has been found to be erroneous. Adequate levels of circulating testosterone are essential for women as well as men, although men need and generally make more. Testosterone supplementations, in the form of creams, which are absorbed through the skin, are very popular. They work so well they are banned in professional cycling. Rather than supplementing testosterone directly in this way, it is better to give your body the raw materials to make its own. Eating lots of fruit and veggies, nuts and seeds, as well as maca, ginger, zinc and selenium will give your body these raw materials.

13. Excess fibrinogen: fibrinogen is a type of soluble plasma protein known as a globulin. Made in the liver, it is essential for coagulation of blood. It interacts with thrombin to form fibrin. It can be a factor in blood clots (thrombosis). Elevation of fibrinogen in the blood is one nonspecific indicator of inflammatory disease. A substance in the body that is essential for coagulation yet can become a risk factor in blood clots, which cause heart attack and stroke. Why it changes from a Jekyll to a Hyde is the subject of continuing research. I predict it will be found that like many unknown causes in the biochemical world, animal "foods" are at the heart of this attack on your heart.[17]

14. Excess homocysteine: Homocysteine is a stress hormone. It is also a general measure of your body's inflammatory status. We all know stress causes tension. It also causes inflammation. Anything that acts as an irritant or stressor to the body is going to increase

homocysteine. Certainly insulting the body with dead decaying flesh that is laced with growth hormone, antibiotics, and pesticides would qualify. Even the so-called "organic" meat is killed on an assembly line, and is therefore shot full of adrenaline and fear vibration. This can only raise stress hormones in your body. The body perceives a threat to itself any time death is introduced in any of its forms. Even cooked food may play a role. Don't worry; you don't have to go raw. Just cook your food as little as possible. You always want your vegetables crunchy. Experiment with more raw dishes. "Don't worry"—is of course good advice to keep stress and stress hormones out of your body.

15. Hypertension, Also known as high blood pressure. OMG, where do I start? I guess, "don't worry" is a good place. We take everything too seriously. Silly humans. Don't we know it will all be over in a few years anyway? Take it light. Stress is a causative factor in high blood pressure, as is salt. Mostly high blood pressure is caused by occluded arteries.[18] As the pathways through which blood travels away from the heart get smaller, pressure is increased, Simple, Simple to fix too, stop ingesting the raw materials that clog your arteries. Decrease LDL; increase HDL. Celery juice has been shown to single-handedly lower BP. Avail yourself of plant helpers to get rid of the blockage you already have. Relax. Enjoy life. Easy.

16. Excess cholesterol: We have already explored this phenomenon in some detail. The body needs cholesterol for many of its functions, and makes its own. No need to worry about not having enough. As with protein, if you are consuming a diet that provides adequate calories to get you through the day you will have

enough cholesterol. Most people have excessive LDL. While this is a cause of heart disease, it is by no means the only one, as we are seeing. We know how to keep excess cholesterol from doing damage. Eat low on the food chain.

17. Oxidized LDL: LDL is in and of itself not bad. The term "bad" cholesterol doesn't really apply. It's only bad when you get too much, which most people do, or when it becomes oxidized.[19] Oxidation is a process that occurs throughout the body. It's easy to visualize its effect because when oxidation occurs on unpainted metal surfaces its called rust. Give rust enough time and it will dissolve the metal completely. This is what is happening in your body. "Free radicals" are atoms with unpaired electrons. An atom can lose electrons through environmental toxins. Toxins can knock off one or more electrons from an otherwise healthy atom. This atom then becomes a free radical trying to steal electrons from other atoms, and damaging them in the process. This is known as oxidation. When LDL becomes oxidized, it becomes even more dangerous. How can we stop LDL from becoming oxidized? Well, we can do our best to avoid toxins. The best plan will be not to allow excess LDL to form. Too much LDL, as we have seen, is a very bad thing. When it becomes oxidized, it's even worse. If we stop eating the foods that cause it to form, we will never have to worry about LDL, oxidized or otherwise. Clean up your diet. Really clean it up. Be happy. Age in reverse.

18. Blood pH in the low or acid range: A body that is too acidic is a sitting duck—waiting for the shotgun of disease to blast it. Like inflammation and high homocysteine, it is a cause within the cause.[20] We must

maintain a near neutral pH at least. If we are eating the age reversing foods and avoiding the acid producing "foods" like wheat and animal products, we can get into an alkaline state. It is highly beneficial to maintain an alkaline state. There is a kit you can buy to find out your urine pH. The darker the color on the test paper, the more alkaline the body. Mine, when I took the test, was so dark it almost looked black. Rock on.

Lack of sleep has now been shown to be a factor in atherosclerosis as well. One scientist I saw quoted on a TV show stated that just one week of disturbed sleep was enough to start a subject on the road to pre-diabetes. Wow. Sleep removes a substance called amyloid beta from the brain. This substance builds up throughout the day. Lack of this removal can predispose one to Alzheimer's and other neurodegenerative conditions.[21] Magnesium is known to improve sleep quality and help those who have trouble falling asleep or staying asleep.

Cell phones emit EMFs (electromagnetic frequencies) that may interfere with sleep patterns. EMFs are also implicated in certain cancers. The take-home message? Don't sleep with your cell phone in your bedroom, as 50% of Americans do.

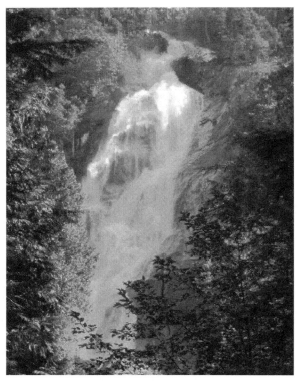

Shannon Falls, Squamish, British Columbia

"No eternal reward will forgive us now for wasting the dawn."

\- Jim Morrison

CHAPTER 13

WATER

N ow, we come to a very important part of the book. We are going to talk about water. What kind of water is best? What kind is aging you at an accelerated rate? While no substance on the planet makes more difference to how we live and age than water, there is much misinformation on it.

We'll start with the worst water and then progress to the best. Short of drinking raw sewage, there is no worse water than bottled.[1] It ranks right behind nuclear power and meat production as an environmental scourge. How? First is the damage it does to our bodies.

The stuff is full of plastic residue, which is not flushed out of the body. Bottled water is always contaminated with BPH, toluene, benzene, and a very long list of other chemicals. See tappedthemovie.com for more of the story. There was a test done on a bottle of a popular water brand that showed huge amounts of toxins in it. The bottle was then left in a car in the sun for an hour, and tested again. The levels of toxins were more than 10 times higher after it had heated up. The plastic gives off more toxins when heated. These bottles are meant to be recycled, and so are very thin and very cheap.

In addition, present in most samples is e coli. Since bottled water is just filtered city water, this is a very profitable venture indeed. Some claim to be spring water, but who's checking. Nobody, I'm not kidding; there is no regulation of this industry. I hope you watch tappedthemovie.com. You may never drink this vile mixture again.

This is an unbelievably profitable business to be in to say the least. It's no surprise that the two largest soft drink companies in the world own two of the best-selling brands. Nestle owns several other brands. It's hard to imagine a more moneymaking business to be in than selling us water. If someone told us 30 years ago that we'd be paying upwards of four dollars a bottle for water, we would have looked at them as if they were crazy.

What's next, bottled air? Don't laugh, there are already a few oxygen bars in Asian cities and even here in America where you can go and breathe some oxygen to help chase away the brain fog from breathing all that polluted air. We may live to see Smartair, or some such. Maybe it will have a name like Mountain Morning or Sea Breeze. I can see it now. There will even be different flavors——smells, maybe some lavender essential oil to calm you, or some peppermint to give you a lift. This could get ugly. I'll bet the same companies that make so much on bottled water will be major players in the bottled air game. See? Living long is not the goal. The buzz is the goal. Who wants to live in a world where you have to pay for air? Or water?

I read in the July-August 2014 issue of the Sierra Club magazine that in China, bags of air from Laojun Mountain are being shipped to Zhengzhou, for citizens of the polluted provincial capital to breathe from. OMG it's starting already.

Indulge me for a moment if you will while I say a word about the cost to our and the planet's quality of life from bottled water. Only 10 per cent of all these millions of bottles are ever recycled. If you do any hiking or kayaking, you've seen many bottles on the trail or river. A huge percentage of them end up in the oceans. Many municipalities routinely dump garbage at sea.

Unlike most plastics, which can survive unchanged for hundreds of years, these thin cheap bottles break down very easily. This is bad news for the ocean. There are two kinds of plankton, zooplankton, and phytoplankton. One is an almost microscopic animal and one a plant. They are the base of the marine food chain. Some marine species eat it directly. Some eat it secondhand by eating other fish, mollusks, etc. Nowadays in most ocean water tested, plastic particles are more numerous than plankton. This means that sea creatures are ingesting massive amounts of plastics and concentrating it in their bodies. This is another reason not to eat fish. Check out the documentary film "Bag It", (bagitmovie.com) for a real appreciation of how far out of hand the plastic problem has gotten.

This all shows how each one of us is either part of the solution or part of the problem. It also shows how, by improving your health, you improve the planet's health. You are helping future generations, which may very well be us in future lives. You are also helping yourself to be less plastic.

This concept of us actually being future generations may be foreign to you. Maybe you believe in a literal hell that we go to if we do bad things. Maybe it will exist. Maybe it will be of our own making. There's a lot to say about water and how we're sucking it out of the ground, from aquifers that do not replenish themselves, at a rate that guarantees they will be depleted at some future point. The world's glaciers, on which much of humanity depends for water, are disappearing at an alarming rate. The population is growing at the unbelievable rate of some 200k people a day.[2] I guess I'd better stick to my subject. I am a victim of my super health. The healthier and cleaner you get, the more you care. Maybe enough of us will start caring to make the difference between losing all this and pulling it out of the fire.

Back to water and how it affects your body. We talked about the worst water. Now, we'll talk about the best. You can purify your water easily and cheaply by simply getting a pitcher water filter, like a Britta or Pur. The one that seems to do the best job is the Zerowater. I use one for traveling. These do not take out all the contaminants, but if money's tight or you need the convenience of something small and easy to use, they beat the hell out of lugging bottles of plastic infested water. You can have water that is much purer than tap or bottled for less than twenty bucks. These filters are a great way to go.

For really purifying your water, a steam distillation system should be in every household. These can be had for a little as $300 and require a bit more work than just pouring water through a filter. They are very easy to use though, only requiring you to fill them up and let them cycle a gallon at a time. Check out waterwise.com. I've had very good service from this company. One of their countertop distillers will serve you for years.

The documentary film "Tapped" compares municipal (city) water favorably to bottled water, because bottled water is full of plastic residue, and chemicals like toluene, etc. Bottled water is also routinely found to be contaminated with fecal coliform and E. coli, just to name a couple of the biological contaminants. City water, being chlorinated, would not harbor these as a general rule. Keep in mind that chlorine as well as the antibiotics in meat and dairy, kills off your friendly bacteria (probiotics).

City water is highly chlorinated and full of lime and worst of all in some cases, fluoride. The idea that fluoride is good for your teeth is absolute rubbish. Most municipalities have by now stopped putting it in water. Fluoride is actually a byproduct of aluminum smelting. Since aluminum toxicity has been linked to Alzheimer's, ADHD, and ADD, it would be interesting to do a study on the municipalities that still use fluoride and its relationship to these afflictions.

Speaking of city water, it is widely regarded that taking a shower in city water exposes you to the same levels of chlorine and other chemicals as you would get from drinking a glass of city water. You also inhale these chemicals in the steam that the hot water produces. Taking a bath in city water is probably even worse because your pores are open from the soaking in hot water and all these chemicals are being sucked into your skin. It's called trans-dermal absorption, and it is the reason testosterone creams and the like work so well. Your skin is a major organ of absorption as well as elimination. The solution? A shower filter. These are very inexpensive. Whole Foods sells one for less than $50. I got mine from waterwise.com for about the same price and have had it for years. You can also get a type that looks like a little basket and hooks over your bath spigot. These are harder to come by but no more expensive. A company called Isabella sells one.

The best water of all is organic water, water that has passed through the cells of a plant. This water will replenish your cellular water.[3] A symptom and a cause of aging is the loss of cellular water. This water is stored inside the cells of the body. Not all water can find its way into the cells. Cellular water depletion is at the heart of aging. As we age, we go from about 80% water to 60% or even less.[4] One place you can readily see this transformation is the skin. As your skin loses cellular water, it thins and dries out. Some cosmetics are formulated to keep the skin not only moisturized, but to seal in cellular water as well. Coconut oil is excellent for this. I've been using it for years as a moisturizer. Another reason the skin loses elasticity and thickness (yes thickness is a good thing when it comes to the skin), is lack of EFAs. Getting plenty of the right fats in your diet is essential to aging well, or aging in reverse.

Cellular water is replenished when you eat plant foods, particularly vegetables and fruits, as they contain the most water. Fresh made or non-reconstituted juices also replenish your cellular water. Even bottled juice, as long as it is not made from concentrate and reconstituted, will replenish your cellular water. My beloved coconut water can also be added to this list. Be aware that cooking more than just a little removes organic water also called "structured" water from vegetables.

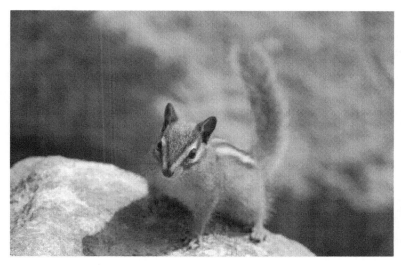

Western Ground Squirrel on the High Note Trail, Whistler
Mountain

"Our bodies are our gardens – our wills are our gardeners."
- William Shakespeare

CHAPTER 14
JUICING AND NUT MILKS

I have been talking a lot about what to stop eating in order to reverse your biological age. Indeed, it seems to be more about what you don't eat than what you do eat, or about exercise, or stress management, or any other factor. That's because the bad 'food' is so much worse than anyone thought, or could even imagine. I hope I've convinced you to see what your life could be without poisoning your body on a daily basis.

Now I'll tell you of some things you can add to your life that will make a dramatic difference in your buzz; the first and most powerful is juicing. So many juicers have been bought by folks with the best of intentions. They start juicing and are disappointed to find out how much work it is and how long it takes. Juicing may be the most important single thing you can do to improve your health. A hassle? No more so than making a meal. You wouldn't start making an elaborate meal when you are pressed for time. Save juicing for when you can devote a bit of time to the process. You can make extra and save some for later as the juice will keep for at least 1-3 days refrigerated.

I will promise you this. As you keep doing it with an eye toward refining your technique, you will cut the time it takes in half or even by two thirds. It's an acquired skill. You will find ways to streamline the process. You will make less of a mess to clean up as you learn how to juice more efficiently. Just stay with it. It will be worth it.

Nothing nourishes your body like vegetable juice. Think about it if you've never contemplated the wonder of juicing. If you drink a glass of carrot juice for instance, you are getting the nutrition of 4 to 6 carrots in that one glass, you'd have to be pretty dedicated to eat that many carrots. All the nutrients in the carrots are much better absorbed in juice form, and you don't have to chew which most people don't do sufficiently anyway. As with all recipes, experiment with different combinations of fruits, vegetables and spices. My favorite is broccoli, celery, red cabbage, cucumber, and beet.

There are two basic types of juicer: centrifugal and masticating. The centrifugal kind is cheaper, unless you get a real heavy-duty one. Several brands sell for $100-$200.[1] If you opt for one of these, be sure to get one that sends the pulp out one side and the juice out the other. These are very easy to use and to clean. They require almost no effort to put the vegetable or fruit through them. The downside with this type is that they are not as efficient at extracting the juice as the heavier, more expensive, and more labor-intensive masticating type.

The centrifugal juicer also doesn't do greens very well. The masticating juicer can juice anything from wheatgrass to potatoes. The masticating juicer juices at a very slow RPM and is much more efficient at extracting all of the juice from the food. The downside is you have to push the food down on to the blades or rollers that are used to separate the juice from the pulp. I have used one for the past 20 years; actually, I'm on my third one now, a Greenstar.[2] It won't last indefinitely, but is an excellent value, and highly recommended. I hope you at least buy an inexpensive centrifugal juicer and start playing around with making the most healthful food on the planet.

If you're pressed for time, or are just not feeling the need to go to the trouble of juicing. I have an easier, though less potent way of doing your body the great favor of ingesting fresh raw veggies. I am, as you may have noticed, unwavering and inflexible on my condemnation of the so-called foods that are

149

hastening you toward an early decline. I am, on the other hand, very interested in making this all doable for you. If it's too inconvenient, you won't do it. An easy and fast way to make an awesome drink, in a word - Vitamix.[3]

No, I'm not being paid for this plug; it's just that I've had such good service out of mine that I must give credit where it is due. I've tried other brands and none are equal to the original high-speed blender. This is a super blender; it differs from the department store variety in that it is much stronger, and will truly liquefy your veggies, fruits, nuts, and seeds. It is probably the best investment you can make in your health. It may seem expensive, but unlike substituting a pitcher-type water filter for a distiller, there is nothing else that can do what a heavy-duty blender does. It will be the best $400 you ever spent and will last for years. They can sometimes be had for as little as $250. Reconditioned Vita mixes are sometimes available on the company website. You will use it every day, I sincerely hope. There is a recipe book that comes with the machine and many more available, but if you experiment, you will come up with your own concoctions. As you know, we are all about doing a diet rich in the wonderful healing properties of fruits, veggies, seeds and nuts. We want to go low carb to a point and take in adequate fat–the right kind that is.

I want to share with you one of the best ideas I ever had - nut and seed milk. I'm not talking about that watery almond or rice milk you buy in the carton. They are usually fortified with the wrong type of calcium. If the calcium contained in the product is calcium carbonate or calcium phosphate, you don't want it. These are rocks. Remember from our talk on dairy, if it's not absorbed, calcium does some very bad things in your body; you cannot absorb this mineral form of calcium. Calcium Ascorbate, Calcium Citrate, and Calcium Piccolinate are the absorbable supplemental forms.[4] I told you earlier in the book how the calcium from dairy is not well absorbed by the body. So where do we get the right kind? Turns out you don't need to supplement Calcium at all. As a word of caution, even the right calcium is only absorbed in the presence of sufficient Vitamin D and magnesium.[5] If you eat the nutrient rich foods suggested here, you will never have to worry and your bones and muscles will have all the calcium they need.

Green veggies have calcium in abundance, and it is the kind your body craves and absorbs. In addition, carrots, oranges, and nuts have lots of calcium too. Sesame seeds and almonds have quite a bit. Chia seeds may be the richest source of all. You need not worry about getting enough calcium if you're eating age-reversal foods.[6] The beauty of not eating all the crap is now you will naturally eat more of the nutrient dense food that make you feel great. So many vegetarians start eating a bunch of starch instead of meat, or almost as bad—soy. You have to be careful with this. We want to replace all the junk with the good stuff.

There is a book, written by a doctor called "Protect your Brain." He states that stroke and Alzheimer's are caused by occluded or partially blocked blood pathways to the brain, and that this blockage is caused by eating animal food–meat and dairy. As prevention, he recommends "healthy whole grains" be part of your diet. Here again, I caution you to listen to some of his message but not to substitute one evil for another. Unlike the doctors who wrote the books on the evils of wheat, he is all about the evils of meat, dairy and eggs. Here again, we can learn from these authors without swallowing their message whole.

So many times, an author will say something like, "So now you know the truth" after expounding on a subject like how bad wheat is for you, for example. You actually won't know at all until you try cutting it out and feel the difference. I am asking you to have the experience of this knowledge...quite different from believing something to be true or being told something, even if it resonates strongly within you, as I hope this does. You must test the validity of any advice or new information. Faith is not needed. Belief is not your friend. Try it and see.

Here is something I really want you to experience–nut and seed milks. Nuts are as close to the perfect food as anything could be. They are full of the beneficial fat that is so lacking in the American diet. They are also one of the best dietary sources of minerals like selenium and zinc, which are also in short supply in most people's diets. They also have lots of the right kind of calcium. The problem is nuts are not well absorbed by most people. Why is this? One reason is that they are often consumed in a highly adulterated state. When they are roasted, or otherwise perverted, they transform from something wonderful to something hideous.

Another reason nuts are not well absorbed is that they are not well chewed. As we discussed before, it is essential to chew all your food well, this is especially true of nuts. They are rather hard and will not be digested if they are not well chewed. I know; chewing nuts well is a lot of work. Your jaws may get tired long before the job is properly done. If you soak them, nuts become much softer, and are not only more easily chewed, but digested as well. Soaking also breaks down any enzyme inhibitors that may be present. Some nuts have a lot of these, particularly almonds.

Almonds really need to be soaked long enough so you can easily pop off the red skin of each one. This makes almonds the most labor-intensive nut to deal with. This is not much of a hassle though. It can be easily done, and like all of these new skills I hope you are learning, like juicing, it just takes a bit of practice to get your technique down. (If the red skin doesn't come off easily, soak them longer) This is the only nut that requires any real work to prepare. I am talking about raw and preferably organic nuts. Raw is the only way to go when it comes to nuts.[7]

Good news; You don't have to chew nuts at all if you have one of the most wonderful inventions known to man...the Vita Mix blender. I have tried others, and found this brand to be the best. It will prove to be worth its weight in revitalized human flesh. This machine will serve you for years, with zero maintenance. I like the simple model (Model 5200) with only a fast and slow switch and a dial to control the speed for the slow setting.

Here is all you do to make fantastic nut and seed milks and even cheeses. Some nuts, like Brazil nuts, Macadamias, and pine nuts do not absorb water, and so, do not need to be soaked. Cashews, being very soft, can be soaked but do not need to be. I find cashews to be the easiest and perhaps the tastiest nut of all. Cashews are a very rich source of tryptophan. Tryptophan is one of the eight essential amino acids. It supplies the raw material to make serotonin, (the "feel good" neurotransmitter) which is so lacking in depressed people. It is also a calming influence on the whole body. Some people take tryptophan in supplement form to help them sleep. Instead of reaching for those antidepressants—start drinking cashew milk.

Here's more good news. The soak water from many nuts and seeds is super probiotic and very tasty. Let's say you're soaking pumpkin seeds. You would know the seeds are ready when the water turns a little green, and has a few bubbles in it. The soak time for nuts and seeds, and the time it takes to make your sauerkraut water from vegetable pulp, also known as rejuvilac, (which we discussed earlier in the book) is temperature sensitive. In other words the warmer the environment, the faster it makes. You can blend the soak water into your nut milk or drink it separately

Now let's make some milk: Let's take the example of cashews. You put a couple of cups or so of cashews in the bottom of your Vita Mix. Cashews, being very soft, could probably be done satisfactorily in a department store blender but will be much more creamy and smooth in the Vita Mix. I hope that you will buy the Vita Mix. Now, you add just enough water to cover the cashews to liquefy them - about a 1:1 ratio. You want just enough water to liquefy. We are always going for maximum agitation. I have found the best way to start the blending process is to start the machine on the low setting with the dial set on a low speed (1-5 on the dial). This process ensures the nuts aren't thrown in pieces to the top of the container. Dial the speed up to 10, and then flip the switch to maximum speed and blend longer than you probably think is necessary (2-3 minutes). We want the nuts completely liquefied. The milk will get a little hot. Your milk can be served hot out of the blender, if you desire. I always have some cold water or coconut water ready to add to it immediately.

Most high-speed blenders use plastic containers, I don't know why. We would ideally like our food never to touch plastic, especially hot plastic. These blenders use a very durable grade of plastic but I can't help wishing they used glass. Having dropped mine a time or two, maybe I should be thanking the manufacturer instead of complaining about the container.

After you add water to reach the consistency you desire, turn the machine back to a low setting and mix it up. More water will make the milk thinner so add less water if you like a milk shake consistency. The high setting is very fast and a little bit loud. Get in the habit of flipping the switch to low and dialing back the speed when you are done blending. When that sucker comes on, set on high-speed, it can freak you out if you're not expecting the noise. That is all there is to it.

I have step-by-step instructions on making nut milk and cheese in the back of the book.

One word of caution. Walnuts, almonds, pecans, hazelnuts and any nut that turns the soak water red or brown must be strained and the water discarded before you use them. The red pigment is an enzyme inhibitor and will inhibit the absorption of many of the nutrients in your nuts. Any nut that will absorb water should be soaked for maximum absorption and ease of digestion.

Using cashews again as an example, wait until you try the nut cheese! All you do is follow the milk recipe without adding water so it is a thicker, pudding like consistency. Put the liquefied nuts in a glass bowl and cover, leaving it until you can taste the cheese has made. Sample it after about 24 hours or so. Like the probiotic soak water, this is a temperature sensitive process. The warmer the ambient temperature in the room, the quicker the cheese will make. The longer you let it set up, the stronger the cheese will be. If you let the cheese sit too long, mold can form on the top. If this happens, no worries, scrape off the top layer and discard, the rest of the cheese will be delicious. You can use this cheese in all sorts of recipes, desserts, drinks, and anything your imagination can conjure up; Super probiotic.

I used to strain all my nut milks because I like them very liquidy. I recently stopped straining them, in favor of just adding water. I'll make a large amount to keep in the refrigerator. If the milk is not strained, it is like a concentrate. You would just spoon some out and add water to taste. This makes it even more convenient. Short of just biting into a piece of fruit, this is the easiest food prep you can imagine. Pumpkin seed milk has become one of my staple foods. I use it to make

155

my amino shakes. Notice I don't say protein shakes, because as I said earlier, it's not protein that builds muscle, its amino acids - the constituent parts of protein.[8] I sometimes add L – Glutamine, L – Carnitine, L – Carnosine, and the branched-chain amino acids - Leucine, Isoleucine, and Valine to the milk. I also add Maca powder,[9] ginger powder and sometimes cinnamon powder. This is my muscle building recovery drink. If you like chocolate milk, add cacao powder. I always add Creatine and vitamin C powder. Another idea for experimentation: I use coconut water to add a bit of sweetness and to add electrolytes. You can also sweeten with maple syrup; grade B is the least processed. You will no doubt, come up with your own ideas. Adding fruit to it also works well.

A tip for experimentation on milks and on recipes in general is to make a large batch and then flavor or spice small bowls or glasses of the recipe with whatever spice or sweetener you want; that way you don't ruin the whole batch if you don't like the result. I hope you will be experimenting a lot with new recipes.

There are many books on raw and vegan recipes. There are also quite a few blender drink recipe books. One comes with the Vita Mix blender. Any recipes that call for milk, cream, or cheese can be made using nut and seed milks and cheeses. Just blend to the consistency you need. You can also use the soak water from nuts and seeds and the probiotic sauerkraut drink in recipes, especially liquid ones. Experiment with the flavors of different nut and seed milks, and tailor them to the recipe you're making.

It's been suggested to me that I should be including more recipes in this book. I have not included very many because there are many books available to turn you on to wonderful raw and vegan recipes. Tribest.com has several, some written by actual raw chefs. As I stated in the beginning of this book, I am sharing with you from my experience. What the hell does a liquidarian know about recipes? I have been on a liquid diet for the past 17+ years. Before that, I was a raw foodist who ate very simply. If I gave you recipes in this book, they would be for dishes I have not tried. I'm not interested in bringing you information I don't know to be true.

Liquid recipes are largely a matter of taste and experimentation. If you make some nut milk and experiment with adding different fruits and anything else that strikes your fancy, you will come up with your own wonderful concoctions. Remember learning new a skill builds new neuronal pathways in your brain. Age your brain in reverse at the same time you get creative with liquid recipes! Recipe books are great to get you started down the road to culinary creativity. Virtually any recipe in a book can be made healthier, and can be tailored to your own tastes through a bit of experimentation. For instance, substituting nut cheeses and milks for dairy products in recipes.

I have found that if you are blending or otherwise liquefying your food, proper food combining matters less. Adding fruit to nut milks seems to work just fine from a digestion standpoint. It's even been said that adding nuts to salad helps you absorb the nutrients in the lettuce better. The main point of food combining is to simplify things for your body. Just be sensitive to what your body is telling you.

One recipe I will share with you is my pomegranate juice smoothie. I make cashew milk or pumpkin seed milk, and add some chia seed milk. (not too much—it's fibrous) Add some blueberries or cherries (fresh or frozen) or any other fruit and blend long enough to liquefy the fruit. Add pomegranate juice and mix on a low setting. I also add vitamin C powder and creatine. The fibrous nature of chia seeds is not a problem for most people, many consider fiber healthy. My body doesn't appreciate fiber. My body would much prefer all my meals were liquid—like juice. You have to make it convenient though, and you can't always juice in the morning. Any way you can get more blueberries and other super fruits into your body is a good thing.

You will find your own favorite recipes with a bit of experimentation. Remember to start blending on low and turn the speed up, then switch to the high setting. Turn the switch back to low after liquefying to avoid the food being thrown up to the top of the blender and to avoid being startled when the machine comes on set on high. Always mix already liquid or powder ingredients on a low speed, to avoid bubbles forming.

One of the best things about quitting the crap food is that you naturally eat a lot more of the truly healthy food. Enjoy this new adventure. Have fun.

Many people feel overwhelmed at learning a completely new way to prepare food. Don't be one of them. Relax into the process of learning new skills and methods.

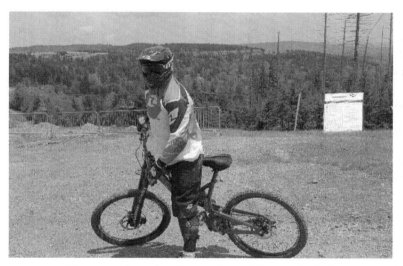

About to drop in, Snowshoe, West Virginia

"Just one smile immensely increases the beauty of the universe."

– Sri Chinmoy

CHAPTER 15
GOT AMPK?

This is a very exciting time to be learning about ways to reverse the aging process. New findings and new answers are coming thick and fast these days. I think I may have just found my answer as to why my LDL cholesterol number is higher than the optimal number of 100 or less. Everything in my blood work, which I did in preparation for this book, was in the optimal range except LDL, which was 126. This number is considered in the "healthy" range by most doctors. Our Dr. Fuhrman has stated that it should be no more than 100.

There are several books in which authors state cholesterol doesn't really matter that much; the body manufactures and needs cholesterol for many of its vital functions. Certainly, it does, but cholesterol does matter—a lot. It's the small LDL (low density) particles of cholesterol that clog your arteries, causing high blood pressure, stroke and the number one killer in developed countries– heart disease.

When my number is above the optimal range, I have to wonder why. I don't eat any of the foods known to raise LDL. Sedentary lifestyle certainly contributes to a high number, but I'm not sedentary. I immediately assumed it must be the red palm oil I consume as a vitamin E supplement. Since palm and coconut oils are the only saturated fats in the vegetable kingdom, I figured this must be the reason, even though I don't use much.

I may now have the real reason. I can thank the Life Extension Foundation once again for hipping me to something very important. They actually did a separate issue of their magazine to alert us to this important new finding. Carbohydrates that cause blood sugar spikes can raise LDL and triglyceride levels in the blood. I have abused carbohydrates in the form of fruit juice for many years. I didn't know any better. Only in the last few years have I been trying to drink a lot less. I say trying because here I come face-to-face with my addiction. I love fruit juice (oops, I said it). I used to practically live on the stuff. It looks like this "carbage" may be the reason for my higher than optimal LDL number.

There is an enzyme in our cells called AMPK which when activated, slows down aging throughout the body. Through a process called "autophagy" it cleans up old/damaged cellular components. In other words, it helps the cells take out the garbage. Toxicity in all its many forms is the cause of aging. We not only get toxins from eating animal "foods", we also reabsorb toxins from cellular debris, and indeed, from any body function that produces waste products that are not removed. This is emerging from the research as a cause of neurodegenerative and other age-related disorders.

AMPK removes the metabolic waste products produced continuously by our cells. This removal process, like virtually every process in the body slows down with advancing age. AMPK, in other words, doesn't work as efficiently on removal as we age. To quote LEF "This dysfunction is so severe that senile cells cannot even commit suicide (apoptosis) because they lack sufficient energy instructions to perform even simple housekeeping tasks. Yet the senile cells emit chronic external signals that create a systemic state of low-level inflammation throughout the aging body."

There's more: "AMPK augments cellular housekeeping. Reduced AMPK signaling on the other hand can exacerbate common problems related to cellular dysfunction like heart failure. Likewise, when type II diabetes manifests, is often caused by a loss of cellular insulin sensitivity. AMPK improves insulin sensitivity." Activating AMPK looks to me like a way to improve virtually every symptom of aging! Definitely gotta get some.

AMPK is found inside every cell. It serves as your body's master regulator. It determines among other things body fat composition and whether cholesterol finds its way into the arteries and stays there, or is metabolized for energy. A quote from that LEF article: "Extensive research shows that by increasing AMPK activation, we can reduce many of the destructive factors of aging, thus enabling cells to return to their youthful vitality."[1]

Here's another: "In preclinical research, enhanced AMPK activity has been associated with a 20 - 30% increase in lifespan, but that's just the beginning of the health benefits conferred by this critical cellular enzyme. Increased AMPK activation has been shown to help reduce fat storage (especially dangerous belly fat), increased insulin sensitivity (due to lower blood glucose), reduce cholesterol/triglyceride production and suppress chronic inflammation. All of these factors underlie the lethal diseases of aging."

The article also states that calorie restriction and vigorous exercise activate AMPK, shrinking body fat stores (especially in the belly region), lowering blood sugar and lipid levels, and producing other beneficial effects that retard the aging process. Lowering blood sugar is a big deal. "Lipid levels" refers to LDL and triglycerides, with must be kept low to protect us from heart disease and all of the other disease systems caused by higher levels. The article further states that when you under eat, you create increased AMPK activity as cells sense a requirement to function more efficiently in the presence of diminished energy (food) intake. However when normal food intake resumes, AMPK activity declines.

So, if you don't exercise vigorously enough to activate AMPK and you are not inclined to do calorie restriction, does that mean you cannot benefit from increased AMPK activity? No. LEF (Life Extension Foundation) to the rescue again. They have just formulated a plant extract supplement to help your body activate and benefit from AMPK. An Asian plant distantly related to the cucumber called G. Pentaphyllum not only activates AMPK, but it also shuttles excess fats into the mitochondria to be utilized for energy and safe disposal. Mitochondria are the energy centers in each of your cells that produce a substance called ATP– your fuel. It therefore increases energy production and decreases LDL and triglycerides in the blood. Sweet. It also increases cellular glucose uptake. This is significant because glucose levels need to be kept in check in our bloodstreams. Like fats (lipids) in our blood, when glucose is not used for energy immediately bad things happen.

Like most – maybe all – body functions, AMPK activation decreases with advancing age. In a study reported in the LEF article, rats supplemented for just four days with a G. Pentaphyllum extract showed, compared with controls: 33% reduced triglycerides, 13% reduced total cholesterol, 33% reduced LDL cholesterol, 20% lower after meal blood glucose. Do you think I'm going to order their formulation immediately? Hell yeah.

The letters AMPK stand for adenosine monophosphate activated kinase. Interestingly, adenosine is the first word in adenosine triphosphate (ATP), the body's fuel supply. All sugars and fats that are burned for energy are first converted into ATP. It would be interesting to take an organic chemistry class to learn more about this connection.

There is another plant compound that increases AMPK activity. It's called trans-tiliroside, and is extracted from plants such as rosehips. It works in a different way than G.Pentaphyllum. It increases the GLUT-4 transporter in cell membranes which helps pull excess sugar out of the blood and into to cells, where it is burned for energy. From the LEF article: "In obese-diabetic mice, supplementation with trans-tiliroside increased fat burning, lowering plasma insulin, lowered free fatty acids, and lowered triglycerides, while increasing levels of andiponectin, a protein hormone that regulates glucose and breaks down fat," Very exciting stuff. The LEF formulation includes both of these miracle plant compounds. Excuse me; I have to go order some.

Since I know I'm not boring you with this incredibly exciting news, one more quote: "When AMPK is activated, cells go into a survival mode, making and storing no new fat, while burning up available fat from storage, pumping glucose in from the blood for additional energy, building new mitochondria for more efficient energy use, and recycling damaged or dysfunctional proteins. These are all beneficial anti-aging mechanisms." Carrying fat around year after year is extremely unhealthy, especially if it is belly fat. Men who carry extra belly fat have a much lower rate of testosterone production than men who are thin, leading to a lowering of libido, decreased energy, increased sarcopenia, and increased risk of heart disease and stroke. If an herbal formulation can help us get rid of fat, it is in and of itself a godsend.

I have experimented for years with different substances, not only omitting some when I read that they are harmful, but adding to my regimen those that seem to show promise in regenerating the body and increasing energy. I'm all about increasing energy. I love having virtually unlimited energy and endurance. I may be about to bump it up to the next level now. I guess I better call LEF back and put a rush on that order. Can't wait to try this stuff. They call it AMPK Activator.

Just so you know; I'm not affiliated with LEF, other than having been a member for over 20 years. I don't get any kickback or compensation from any of the companies I recommend in this book. If any of them want to give me a discount though, I would be open to that...

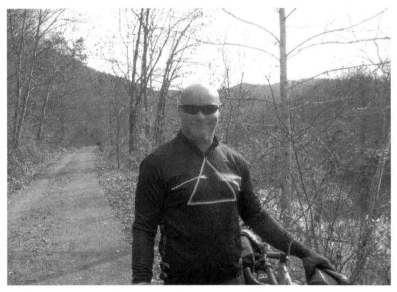

Riding the Greenbrier River Trail, West Virginia

"Persistence guarantees that results are inevitable."

\- Paramahansa Yogananda

CHAPTER 16
TRANSITION—NEW THOUGHTS

Several benefits go way beyond what these new foods and recipes do to reverse your age. Research is showing us that learning new skills builds new neural pathways in the brain. Learning new skills regenerates your brain. It even causes the brain to grow new cells. Learning new skills increases "neuroplasticity"—the brains flexibility and ability to learn and adapt. Something most of us loose more and more as we age.

Another benefit is that now you have something interesting and truly healthy to bring to any dinner party. Sometimes, you have to bring your own food anyway. Don't think of this as rude; on the contrary, now you have something to share, something to be excited about, something that shows the reason for the change they see in you. Any time you don't eat what somebody else is eating, you are doing them a service no one else will probably ever do them. You are showing them a whole other reality as it were. As they observe you aging in reverse, they may very well be motivated to make some changes themselves. What better service could you be to someone than this? Far from putting a perceived wall up between you by not doing what they are doing, you are showing them something amazing, something unique. Remember, most people are under the impression that age reversal is impossible. You could open their eyes just by doing what you're doing and sharing your experience.

I notice whenever I am not eating what is offered it opens a conversation. They usually ask "why?" and I have a chance to share something no one else may ever share with them.

Usually, the topic is dropped; we talk about something else, no big deal. Food is charged with such emotion. This is due to the media and our upbringing and conditioning. Let's take the charge out of it and reclaim our free will.

"You don't have to eat what they serve–don't believe a word, money talks, but you don't have to listen." This is a line from a song I wrote. This is a very beautiful world we live in, but it's getting less beautiful by the day, and so is your body. Turns out the reasons for both are poor choices, uninformed choices, untested hypotheses, and a lot of bad information. We are being sold daily many bad ideas. So much of what we have come to believe about food is false, and extremely detrimental to us and to this planet. Actually, of course, the planet doesn't care. It will go on as it has with or without us. What a shame though that by the same methods we use to destroy our own health, we destroy the health of this ecosystem. So many innocent bystanders are being savaged.

I just read a magazine article about the last bighorn sheep left in an area of Wyoming. He had become habituated to people, people were feeding him candy bars, hamburgers, and God knows what else, and it killed him. I've actually seen people feeding bologna sandwiches to deer. This is further proof that we are not omnivores. Even herbivores can eat meat without dying immediately. Nevertheless, it will kill them eventually, just as it will kill us.

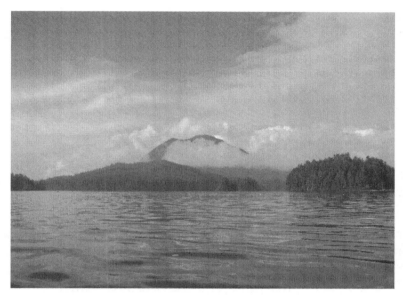

Island Hopping in a sea kayak, Clayoquot Sound

"Insanity: Doing the same thing over and over again and expecting different results."

\- Albert Einstein

CHAPTER 17
DETOXIFICATION

I must say again at the beginning of this chapter that all animal bodies, ours included, have evolved no efficient pathways for ridding the body of toxins. This is the reason you get so much toxicity from eating animal "foods". So how do all the toxins come out? How can we help them come out? The word "detoxification" has become such a buzzword these days. I guess we intuitively know that these bodies are full of toxins. I could go on and on about what's in there, but I'd only be scratching the surface.

The caustic irritants in the average diet keep us constrained by "what happens." When you constantly ingest the wrong kind of carbohydrate, antibiotics in the meat and dairy, growth hormones, pesticides in meat, eggs and dairy, and soyatoxin, just to name a few, not to mention the adrenaline and fear of slaughtered animals, you cannot possibly feel peaceful.

When you have these toxins circulating throughout the body and brain, you are at the mercy of circumstance. Let me explain. When toxins are in circulation, you are in a state of heightened agitation. All it takes is somebody pulling out in front of you in traffic, or some small setback in your life to cause you to become angry or agitated. Some people go through life in what you might call a "generally pissed off" state. Most of us are one small circumstance away from anger. Notice how some people (maybe even you) can be happy and smiling one minute, then due to something somebody says or some small thing that happens, are now feeling anything but happy.

Spiritual evolution is all about not being afi
circumstance. Rising above circumstance—being "in t   ⌐.iu
but not of it". We do not have to be affected by what happens
in our everyday lives. People meditate for years to achieve this.
I have noticed in my friends who do meditate that it doesn't
always work. If they were to clean out the caustic irritants from
their diet, I guarantee they would have a lot more success in
creating peace and tranquility in their lives. Please do not
believe me. I could never communicate to you what this is
about. You must experience it for yourself to understand the
difference between eating toxins on a daily basis and cleansing
them out of the body for good.

There are many ways to detoxify. You can even do an
intravenous "chelation," where you sit and let a chemical flow
into your arm that chelates, or pushes toxins out of their hiding
places in the body. Many people have benefited by doing the
"Master Cleanse" fast, where you eat nothing and drink only
water with cayenne pepper, lemon juice, and maple syrup. The
problem is that when most folks finish the fast they go back to
their old ways. It is not easy on the body to detoxify, no matter
how you do it. This is because it has not evolved with all these
toxins, and has evolved no mechanism for getting rid of them.
It causes a lot of "wear and tear" on the body to detoxify.

As I said earlier, glutathione is depleted when detoxing,
which is significant because without it in abundance you are
more susceptible to the damage these toxins cause. Case in
point, glutathione; while it's produced in the liver, it also
protects the liver. A company decided adding N-acetyl cysteine
(NAC), a precursor to glutathione, to the over-the-counter pain
medication acetaminophen would be a good thing, because this
drug does liver damage, but some people feel they need to take
it to get through the day. The FDA told them it would have to
be approved as a completely new drug, which is so expensive

that this company had to give up the idea. So now, no one can benefit from the combination. Many livers will pay the price. Anyway, depletion of glutathione is just one toll that detoxing takes on the body.

So how in the world are we supposed to detox? Very slowly. In fact, you don't have to worry so much about detoxing—just stop retoxing. Like that word? I made it up. If we stop putting all this junk in, the body will clean itself out––to a point. You can help it greatly in this. I'm here to tell you; the difference is night and day between a toxic body and a clean[er] one. We want to reach a state I call "functionally clean," where the body is by no means completely clean—if that were even possible, but has reached a point in the cleansing process where it functions at a whole 'nother level. You get "over the hump" so to speak. You no longer get irritable and tired when you are hungry. You no longer feel that false hunger that you used to feel and that you used to allay the symptoms of by eating. You start feeling amazing, compared to the way you used to feel—much more focused and energized. There is much more to come as you continue to cleanse, but you are to the point where you are feeling the difference.

The body has three ways of eliminating toxins: pooping, peeing, and sweating. Some comes out in the breath also or hadn't you noticed? That's why "morning breath" is so bad in most people. The body tries to detoxify at night while you sleep. Actually, it tries to detox any time it gets some breathing room. This is why we get irritable when we are hungry. The body starts flushing toxins when it isn't busy with digestion. It's as if our organs are busy little animals. When they get a break from digesting, they start cleaning house. This is why fasting is such an effective cleanser. Couple that with some other detox protocols, which I'll get to in a minute, and you'll have a great way to get the lead out. Beware though, if this happens too fast you will feel it. What is happening is the toxins are coming out of suspension and into circulation. Detoxing is a two-stage process. First, you have to get the toxins moving, and then you have to keep them moving out of the body. When you do the fasting thing or anything like apple, or citrus juice, or some other detoxing juice in enough quantity, the toxins are mobilized. Remember, not eating for a while starts the detox process too. The more toxic your body is the quicker you get cranky and irritable. No wonder there's so much road rage out there. Headaches are a symptom of detox as well. In fact, all headaches are caused by toxicity except the ones that result from a bump on the head. It takes at least three weeks to a few months to start the actual starvation process.

Some people who are lost in the woods or at sea have died of supposed starvation in a few days, even though they had plenty of water. What does this tell you? For one thing, if you expect to die, you will. More profoundly, these folks were overwhelmed by their toxins. Their toxins were really mobilized. This would no doubt lead to all kinds of bad decisions too. Therefore, detoxing has to be done carefully. Not that it will kill you, but why feel all grumpy and low energy?

Here I must warn you that just quitting the foods I'm asking you to give up can also cause you to go into detox mode. These so-called foods are so heavy and hard to digest, so full of toxins that stopping them is almost like a fast. This gives you some insight into how toxic that body of yours really is. Thank God you found this book.

Now to tell you how to reverse that trend and add years to your life, and life to your years. You do more pooping, peeing, and sweating. Pooping gives the most bang for the buck; you just need to do more of it. How? Drinking more water is a good start. I had a woman come to me referred by a friend who I had helped, who had very low energy. She said she wanted to go to bed at 10 in the morning, and not in a good way. I started by asking what she ate for breakfast. The answer, a whole-wheat English muffin with peanut butter and coffee. "How often do you poop?" I asked. "Less than once a day" was her answer. "Can you help me?" she asked. "Oh yeah, we gotta get you pooping in the morning."

Here's my recommendation: as soon as you get up, drink as much as you can handle of some kind of juice. At least a quart and more if you are able. Any kind of 100% juice will do. Fresh vegetable would be best, but make it convenient for yourself. Then go sit on the toilet and do some deep breathing. Several things will happen, all of them wonderful. You will have some good carbohydrates to give you energy, you will for once be hydrated in the morning, you will have the antioxidants in the juice working for you, and drinking a large amount of liquid stimulates peristalsis, to get things flowing.

"Nothing will come out," she said. I said, "Just try it." The process worked. She called a couple of days later to tell me how energized she felt, and to ask if it was normal to go several times a day and have it be liquidy and smell really bad. I said, "You go girl." The smell was all that toxic build up that was making her tired. Those toxins are no small matter. They are a major part of what ages you. If you clean them out, you will age in reverse. Of course, you have to stop putting them back in too.

Yes, I know fruit juice is too high in sugar to be a regular part of your diet. Right now though, you need all the help you can get. You need the carbs that fruit juice provides, as well as the antioxidants, vitamins and electrolytes that fruit juice contains. Fruit juice works well as a sports drink also. The sugar in it will not do its damage if it is needed immediately for energy.[1] You can dilute fruit juice with water to taste if you like.

I've also worked with people who have the seemingly opposite reaction– feeling worse instead of better. I was able to motivate them to make the changes, as I hope I will with you, but it was too much too fast. They failed to keep the toxins that were being released from their hiding places moving out of the body.

Not that you need to taper down your eating of crap. In AA, they don't tell alcoholics to drink less. They tell you to stop. Alcohol, I recently found out, is the only drug you can die from detoxing. It's that poisonous. Even heroin won't kill you trying to kick the habit. You will get very sick (cold turkey), but you won't die.[2]

A friend has finally quit drinking. It was a long hard road. He was the one that told me how if you've been alcoholic long enough, you need to kick under supervision, because people have died suddenly while detoxing. There is a certain way you have to do it.

There is a certain way that's easy and painless to kick the junk food too. Here it is, enemas. No, it's not quite that simple, but it is that easy. I have encountered some resistance on this point; imagine that! Some folks flat out refuse to even try it. I can usually get them to try it eventually.

I guess it would be helpful to share my story about cleansing. I know my case is not typical because I started at such a young age. I was therefore not nearly as toxic as the people I have worked with and am working with now—you. Nevertheless, the process is the same and the results are just as rewarding. I first heard the word "enema" from some hikers I met on the Pacific Crest Trail in California in 1975. They were also some of the first vegetarians I ever met. They were talking about fasting and doing enemas and how awesome it was. I said, "Not me," but the seed was planted. I did resonate with the idea of cleaning the stuff out, but didn't figure I had much to clean out. How wrong I was. Finally, a year or so later, I got a hold of the classic book "Become Younger" by Dr. Norman Walker. The author made a convincing case that a lot of residue from all that horrible food I used to eat was in the colon, causing "autotoxification," in other words, reabsorbing. Yuck. Many of the toxins I'd consumed were still in there doing more damage; Oh my God, I got the picture. Time to do this. But I've got to put something where?

I bought an enema bag and realized that the part that goes in where the sun doesn't shine was not any bigger than a pencil. I can do this. I can't say I enjoyed my first one, but it wasn't too bad. I have no pleasurable sensations from the penetration, but it's really no big deal. It is kind of cool to feel the water going in. Kinda puts you in touch with your body.

Your colon is a very large organ, and makes up a large part of your digestive plumbing. I've read that it is one of the very first organs to form in the developing fetus. It's a core organ, one that has been very badly abused. As I said earlier, colon cancer is now the #3 killer in this country. It has risen rapidly up the charts. You might say with a bullet, like the hit song chart. This ain't no song though. This is a big deal. Again, I will say that this is actually good news. So much of what happens health wise, we feel powerless about, like genetics. Forget it. You hold the power. Enemas are one way to connect with your power. Get in touch with your unlimited soul. Find the freedom within this illusion.

So much of our lives we have felt disempowered. No more. The choice is yours. Declare your independence from convention. Try something new. Let a little water in. It's all in your mind. If you have some resistance to this, tune in to the heart and let the water flow. You will be glad you did. There is nothing unnatural about enemas. Yogis in India long ago learned to do this without an enema bag, by sitting in water and using the abdominal muscles to bring the water in. I haven't tried that. This ain't ancient India. I don't know of any water that would be warm enough that I'd want to do that with, but it shows what's possible. The Essenes also have a technique to bring the "angel of water" into your temple. Water is sacred in many cultures; sadly, ours is not one of them. It's sacred to me, and I use it in my temple (body).

A concern I've heard is that taking enemas and colonics will make the colon lazy, or even make you dependent on them in order to go. Nothing could be further from the truth. I've found that they do nothing but help. I started doing them in 1976. I've had hundreds of enemas and colonics. I have my own colonic machine. I had a woman a few years ago tell me that she asked her doctor about colonics. I was like, "Oh great, what did he say?" "He said they can be habit forming and that you don't need them." I told her to ask him if he'd ever even seen a colonic machine. People are so quick to weigh in on subjects they know nothing about.

A woman in our local raw food group leant me a book by a Russian guy that has a chapter about a girl who was breatharian. He had stayed with her and was interested in her non-eating state, though he had no aspiration of doing it himself. I must admit I'm intrigued too, though my liquidarian diet is a far cry from not taking nourishment at all. If you're interested, check out a book called "Living on Light". There are two accounts of breatharian women in "Autobiography of a Yogi" by Paramahansa Yogananda. A great book that certainly changed my life.

Anyway, what I started out to say is, this guy was a big proponent of enemas, but stated that he'd never had a colonic, and that they could be dangerous. Say what? Why say anything if you don't know what you're talking about? I'm not poo-pooing someone who doesn't agree with me here. I'm just tired of so many people talking about things they have no clue about. I am being very careful in this book not to do that. If I cite a fact that I don't know from experience to be true, I'll qualify it with something like "the research shows", or "I've read." Ok I feel better now. All this to say, please don't listen to folks who don't know and have not experienced. Jimi Hendrix's first record was titled "Are you Experienced?" that really is the question, isn't it? Especially in the topics discussed in this book. I am of no service to you if I'm just another talking head. So now, you know enemas are awesome, right. No, you have to experience it for yourself. Start out slow, with half a bag of water (about a quart) and have fun.

Now what about colonics? A colonic is like a series of enemas. It's like just relaxing and letting the water in and out. There are two basic kinds now: the open system and the closed system. The open system is fairly new. I still prefer the old closed system. I hope you get a chance to try them both.

In the closed system, when you are full enough, you tell the therapist (operator) to flip the valve and release the water. There is a glass section of the machine where you can see what comes out. Fascinating—no, really! The process is repeated until you feel like you're done, or time runs out. You can usually get about eight or so fills. The newer open system has no therapist involved. The water flows in continuously through a very small rectal tube. When are ready, you release it on your own. If you have to urinate, you can just let it go. On the closed system, you can't (without making a mess).

Neither comes with any risk whatsoever. If anything had ever happened accident wise with colonics, the media would be all over it. We would surely hear about the alternative therapy that was dangerous. The concern would be that it could rupture the colon. This is impossible because the tube would be blown out of you before anything like that could happen.

The drawbacks to colonics are that they're pricey–$70-$90 a session most places. You also have to go somewhere to do it. I recommend getting your own colonic machine if you can afford it. You can get a closed system for about $5,000.[3] The open system is about twice that. Though an operator is involved when you have a closed system treatment, you can easily do it all yourself. I've given myself hundreds (maybe that's a bit of an exaggeration).

Why so many you might ask? The colon can hold a lot of stuff. I used to ask my first colon therapist if I was almost clean yet. He would never give me a straight answer. That's like asking if I'm almost enlightened. Silly. Just keep on cleansing. The good news is that the more you cleanse the better you feel. I'm ok with feeling better and better. I can deal. This is such a fun journey; I don't need to "get there."

For most folks, enemas work just fine. I hope you do try colonics, but you really don't need to. You gotta work the enemas though. Why wouldn't you? I know, you don't like the idea. Just try it is all I can say. I had, as I've shared, a real aversion to it at first too. I feel ya. Just try it. You have nothing to lose but years of accumulated sludge.

I am asked sometimes if colonics go "higher" than enemas. In other words, do colonics fill you up more? There is no partition in the colon. In anatomical drawings, you will see the different parts of the colon named. There is no divider in there, so if you want to take more water, just pop it in. Speaking of anatomy drawings, I've read that nobody's colon really looks like the ideal, except maybe some kids that were raised on raw food. I don't know this to be true.

My first colon therapist had a chart on the wall showing three configurations the colon can take. One showed a narrowing of the transverse colon. One a prolapsing where the colon droops and one a large bulge at the sigmoid colon. This is the last part just before the rectum. This deformity is quite common, because when you have to go and don't, the peristaltic movement only goes one way—down.

One way our colons differ from the large intestine of omnivores is that they're flexible. It can end up very big down there at the bottom. How many folks have you seen who are not that fat, or maybe not fat at all, who have a large paunch down low? I once went to a friend's graduation from yoga teacher's training. One by one, the students got up, hugged the instructor, and got their certificates. They were in profile to me and I couldn't help but notice these beautiful young girls had the "pooch" down low. Some more than others, but they all had it.

My first colon therapist said he could tell that I had a narrowing of the transverse colon due to stress. Maybe. I'm sure it's been pushed back into shape now. That's one reason to go for bigger fills.

Before I am done with the colon rap, I want to stress again, how different our colons are from other animals. It's proportionately longer and a lot fatter (wider volume) than the large intestine of other animals. It's very flexible, not like the large intestine of an omnivore at all. As I said before, the colon absorbs all our liquid. Reading the health books early on, none ever stated that the colon is the organ that assimilates all our liquids. They talked about how the colon was a repository for waste that the body was trying to get rid of, and how we are always reabsorbing these toxins. They talked about how no animal food has fiber, and that most of the foods we think have fiber are really just more sludge. Wheat gluten (glue) is just as bad as the animal food in this regard.

When I went to massage school and took anatomy classes, I learned why it's such a big deal that the colon is harboring old waste, and why it's so adept at causing the body to reabsorb toxins. It's because every bit of water absorbed by the body comes through the walls of the colon. Unlike any other animal, instead of a large intestine, we are blessed with a colon. This wonderful reservoir and bringer of liquid to the whole body is unique in the animal kingdom.

Never before have people been exposed to such an unbelievable array of pollution, additives, antibiotics, radiation, the list could go on and on. Immediately following the Fukushima earthquake, fish started to be caught off the coast of California with high concentrations of radioactivity. No fish is safe to eat anymore. The government has set standards for the level of mercury we can safely be ingesting on a daily basis. There is actually no safe amount of mercury.[4]

Cilantro is a miracle detoxing food. Cilantro can actually remove radioactive isotopes from the body.[5] I've never read about anything else except iodine that could do that. It has been used to clear mercury from the body. When we have our mercury amalgam fillings removed, we are spared the daily ingestion of mercury every time we chew. Removal does nothing to get rid of the mercury already stored in the body. Cilantro to the rescue. It is a wonderful addition to salads, or any other dish you are making. It can also be juiced and added to any vegetable juice concoction. Many people add it to their breakfast smoothie, just by dropping some leaves in while they are making it. I hope you will experiment with this wonderful blessing.

You may think so-called organic meat is better than the feedlot, chicken house variety. Certainly organic meat is a little better, but it will destroy your health just the same. Don't believe me? Stop eating it for six months, then eat meat, organic or otherwise, and see what happens. Your body will talk to you. Your body will let you know it is none too happy. The body is very wise; it's our minds that need work.

Wild game is not safe either. I watched a show about California condors. Many of them are dying as a result of eating "gut piles" left by hunters after they field dress their deer. The condors are dying of lead poisoning because when bullets hit meat they fragment and leave lead in the deer meat. The hunters who eat the meat ingest lead too. This is another example of how animals get revenge on us for killing and subjugating them. All right, let's get to the good news. If you stop eating this stuff not only will you age in reverse, you will attain a level of health and happiness that you cannot now imagine, in ways you cannot now imagine.

One thing I have noticed is that I am much more resistant to heat and cold than I used to be. I've always enjoyed cold weather but heat is not my favorite. Two years ago, I was riding my mountain bike in the teeth of a Georgia summer. I was clawing my way up a rocky little climb, pouring sweat out of every pore. I call it multitasking–taking a ride and having a shower at the same time. Yes, it was hot; it occurred to me though, I didn't feel that hot. I certainly was, but it wasn't bothering me as it used to. It wasn't slowing me down as it used to. My intuition told me that I had reached the next level.

This is one of the hallmarks of aging. Older people can't handle the cold anymore, and move to Florida or Arizona, or some other warm place; of course, when it gets too hot, they can't handle that either. Please don't take my word for any of this. Find out for yourself how age reversal works. Feeling better and better instead of worse and worse can be attained so easily. There is no need to trash our bodies on a daily basis, at the same time we trash this planet.

I could tell you that having read this book; you now know how what you call food has been aging you. Of course, you don't know yet; you have to experience it for yourself.

It's also a good idea to minimize the toxins you encounter on a daily basis. Your sense of smell will guide you. As you get cleaner and healthier, the smell of toxins will bother you more and more. If you choose to stay in a toxic environment, you will notice that you smell them less and less. Smelling them less and less is an example of your body supporting your freewill. I have always had a serious aversion to cigarette smoke, which severely curtailed my music career. My body was very wise in not allowing me to breathe cigarette smoke. Now, it has been shown to be full of cadmium and up to 44 different carcinogens.[6]

Just keep an open eye toward any way to avoid toxins. You are going to get a first-hand view of what toxins do to you as you eliminate them. As you detoxify, just by changing your diet for the better, you may feel irritable, fatigued, cranky or any other adjective that describes being low-energy and generally pissed off. Women will have an easier time with this than men will. Women are usually a lot less toxic. One reason is they tend to eat less. The main reason for women's longer life span is that for all of their childbearing years, they had a monthly flush of toxins. Yes, the menstrual cycle is a good thing for detoxing. Men do not benefit from a similar flush. This explains why women often feel all of the aforementioned negative reactions to cleansing at this time of the month. As you get cleaner, your periods become easier and easier. You will flow much less blood and have none of the negative emotional and physical pain you used to experience. The more toxic a woman is, the tougher her period. This toxicity is why the blood often smells bad.[7]

This is the same reason the food smells so bad when it comes out of your body. Your body is much more toxic than you can now imagine. The good news is, it doesn't have to be this way. As you clean out this filth from your body, you will start to feel clearer, happier, and so much more peaceful than you ever thought possible.

I want to tell you two stories I read early on in my quest for knowledge about health and regeneration. The lady who coined the term "rejuvilac" to describe probiotic drinks, and who brought knowledge of wheatgrass and sprouts to the modern age was one Ann Wigmore. She wrote a book called "Be your own Doctor" which was very influential. She was very sick when she found these alternative ways to regain health. Subsequently she ate only raw foods, juiced, fasted, and took colonics and enemas on a regular basis. In her later years, Ms. Wigmore's hair changed from gray to her natural brown in the course of her healing. She aged in reverse. Tragically, she died in a fire at The Hippocrates Health Institute, which she founded.[8]

The other story was related by Dr. Norman Walker, who invented the first juicer. He was also an influential health pioneer. He founded a health institute outside of Phoenix, Arizona, where he would take people diagnosed with terminal diseases and bring them back to health. Many terminal cancer patients were cured. He preferred to treat people before they were ravaged by chemotherapy and radiation, but would generally take anyone who showed a willingness to embrace the changes he outlined.

A woman was carried in and set before him for her entrance interview. She weighed about 60 pounds, skin, and bones. Doctors had given up on her after chemo and radiation failed to have an effect on her cancer, which had metastasized throughout her body. She was in such rough shape, Dr. Walker informed her there was nothing he could do, and it was time to make her transition. She looked at him and pleaded to be accepted saying, "I want to live." He shook his head and restated there was nothing he could do for her.

She then told him she had to live, and was determined. He told her that for someone in her condition to pull it out of the fire would be 1 in a million shot. She looked at him and said, "I'm that one in a million." This moved the doctor, and he relented, saying, "You have to do everything I tell you to do." She agreed, whereupon Dr. Walker informed her that she would have nothing but carrot juice until he said differently, and that she would have colonics twice a day.[9]

To make a long story short, he kept her on nothing but carrot juice for three years. After a month or so, she was able to walk to the bathroom by herself, something she hadn't done in years. Within a few months, she was walking outside, enjoying the fresh air. After her first year, she was up to 120 pounds, putting on muscle on nothing but carrot juice; So much for the myth that you need massive amounts of protein to build muscle.

Look how much muscle cows have eating nothing but grass. These stories illustrate the body's amazing ability to regenerate, to rebuild, and to rebound. All we have to do is stop the war. All we have to do is stop the killing. We are at war with our own bodies. We are killing ourselves, and taking the rest of the animal kingdom with us. When we stop the war with our own bodies, we will stop fighting.

As I've said before, I don't call what I do anti-aging. I don't want to be anti-anything. I'm not fighting. Anti-aging implies a future event; it implies an extension of the lifespan which given today's world situation may not even be a good thing! I'm about the buzz; the here and now. It's not about the future. It's about the present. It's the gift I give myself, and thereby, the rest of humanity. It's my contribution to this beautiful world. Let's call it youth extension, or since most of us have lost our youth, youth reclaiming.

Don't let anyone tell you regeneration can't be done. Remember, people are very quick to weigh in on things they know nothing about, whatever professional title they may hold notwithstanding. Yes, it goes against conventional wisdom that you can reclaim your youth. If you haven't had the experience, you could not possibly know what age reversal is about.

In our quest to age in reverse, it may be helpful to quantify exactly what aging is. Certainly, one cause and hallmark of aging is toxicity. As we age, we collect toxins, which accelerate all aging processes. Our bodies haven't really evolved ways to eliminate and cope with these toxins. Nowadays we have many more toxins, both in variety and volume than we ever had to deal with before as a species. This leaves us ill equipped to handle these insults to our health, longevity, and overall enjoyment of life. It's been said we consume and are exposed to more toxins in a day than our grandparents had to deal with in a year. The variety and complexity of toxins today make this comparison almost meaningless.

Another hallmark of aging is the body slowing down its manufacture of hormones, cofactors, neurotransmitters, etc. Testosterone and serotonin are cases in point. We talked about glutathione earlier. You'll recall that it is depleted in times of stress, which for many people, is all the time. We can supplement glutathione, testosterone, estrogen, serotonin, and other substances directly, but this prompts the body to stop making its own, or at least slow down the manufacture of these substances.

This is not what we want. Rather than supplementing these substances, it is far better to give your body the raw materials to make its own. (Like NAC in the case of glutathione, and tryptophan with seratonin) This lack of raw material is a big reason the body doesn't make enough. Another reason we don't make enough is the general lack of vigor and vitality that occurs with aging. By revitalizing the body, through the mechanisms we have discussed, especially not putting junk in it, these processes will start to work a lot better.

Neurotransmitters work the same way. This is why antidepressants are so popular these days and one reason they are so dangerous. Serotonin, the feel-good neurotransmitter, so lacking in people who are depressed, is artificially induced by antidepressants. The problem is antidepressants come with a host of side effects, such as low libido, lethargy, and irritability. Another problem with antidepressants is that your body stops making serotonin naturally. So, instead of very little serotonin, you have virtually none when you try to quit the drug. This is why they tell you that you can't get off antidepressants without a long tapering process.

I once met a woman through an online dating service who was depressed. She had the usual stresses; raising three children, dead-end job that she hated, not enough money...you know what I mean. She had been on Prozac for well over 10 years, and was experiencing all the side effects. She was desperate to get some energy back and to feel good again. She was so desperate to feel something positive, she asked her doctor to please take her off this medication. He outlined a plan that would take months or possibly years to achieve. He advocated reducing the dosage and replacing it with other drugs.

When she asked my opinion, I suggested stopping immediately despite what the doctor said. She questioned my judgment, until I asked her the question, "Is this the same doctor who put you on that stuff in the first place?" That got her thinking. I suggested replacing this drug with something I read about called SAM-e.[10] SAM-e is a naturally occurring substance the body makes which is severely depleted in many people. Like many substances the body makes, you make less of it as you age. It always pays to stay abreast of the latest research findings, when it comes to health. Even if you are the picture of health, you may be able to help someone less fortunate or careful than yourself.

She told me about her doctor's stern warning that to abruptly stop Prozac would be extremely dangerous. I said it would be easy enough to start taking it again if what I suggested didn't work. This made sense to her and she decided to try the SAM-e. She called me a week or so later, feeling amazing, with more energy than she'd had in years. She also said that her arthritis in both knees had vanished. When she related this, I was reminded I had read that SAM-e also helps with arthritis and joint issues.

The moral of this story is we must take responsibility for our own health; we must find our own answers. Do not fault the doctors for not knowing about stuff like this. They are products of their training. They are medical doctors, taught to match a drug with a symptom. Some do stay abreast of other therapies not covered in their medical training, but this is extremely rare, I have found. Dudes are busy, give them a break. Just don't expect them to know much about alternative therapies.

While we're on the subject of serotonin, I might add that your body also tends to stop making serotonin when getting hits of it from stimulation by foreign substances, like alcohol or drugs. This is one reason alcoholics have very little interest in things like sex. Even something like buying a new car doesn't give them the same high it might the rest of us. They need the alcohol to release serotonin. As you continue to use alcohol and drugs, this only gets worse and worse.

This brings me to something I would like to tell you a story about - vaccinations. No doubt, you have had your share, as I have. The story goes like this. I met a woman at one of our raw food meet ups, who was a major crusader against vaccinations, especially mandatory ones. She has a son who is well over 30, yet still lives with her, unable to keep a job other than temporary day labor he picks up.

She said he, as a young child, was about to be enrolled in school, whereupon she was informed he could not be enrolled until he had all his vaccinations. She, being into all things natural, had never given him any. She tried to fight this, but was overruled, and even threatened with prosecution. She relented, and he got his shots. The child was a normal bright, happy young man who was just starting to read and who spoke well. His development was in every respect normal and healthy. As soon as he got his injections, she said, he changed dramatically. He stopped talking for years. He was severely learning-disabled and dyslexic. Now, she will probably have to care for him until she is no longer able to do so. She kicks herself every day for going against her intuition.

I have one question for people who insist that every child be vaccinated because theirs is. If you believe so much in immunization, then your child is safe, right. What does it matter if mine is not?

Vaccination is credited with eradicating diseases like tuberculosis. I read that tuberculosis was on the way out anyway. Polio is another possible case in point. Diseases like this are dangerous for a time, and then disappear. There was no vaccination involved in the eradication of the black plague, or the influenza pandemic that killed so many people during World War I. These pathogens ran their course and disappeared. Smallpox killed more Native Americans during the white man's expansion than guns, and then faded into obscurity. This list could go on and on.[11]

There is major controversy on the point of whether vaccinations eradicated smallpox or polio. I am not stating facts I know to be true here. I am drawing on reading I've done. I don't claim to know one way or the other. Certainly many diseases that have disappeared after killing large numbers of people have died out without the help of vaccines.

So, if you've already had your shots, what is the benefit of me elucidating on this point? It is a cautionary note. My 84-year-old father used to get the flu shot every year even though the shots only cover one or two strains of influenza. There are generally new strains every year, so flu shots can be very ineffective. It was recommended by his doctor that he get one because the elderly can be severely affected by the flu. Therefore, he did. My mother on the other hand would have none of that. One year, right after his shot, he got the flu. He has since discontinued flu shots and hasn't been sick since.

If you keep your immune system strong and vibrant, you will shrug off invading pathogens. Remember, pathogens of all kinds mutate because of the host they land on. In other words, if they find a favorable place to grow and proliferate, they will. If your immune system is strong, they will not.

All we can do as adults is thank our lucky stars we didn't develop autism from immunization and hope the mercury in vaccinations doesn't affect us too adversely. Mercury is, after all, toxic in any amount, yet it is used as a preservative and carrying agent in vaccinations to this day.[12] It is also routinely still put into people's mouths as a cavity filler.[13]

I once had a very interesting experience before I had my three fillings removed. It was at a health Expo, visiting a booth selling a mercury chelation product. The proprietor had a machine that measured the amount of mercury in your mouth. Intrigued, I took the test. He had me bite down on a mouthpiece while a needle on a gauge gave a reading of how much mercury was present in my mouth. He remarked on my low level, and I told him I only had three fillings. He then had me chew gum for a couple of minutes, spit it out, and bite down on the mouthpiece again. I was amazed to see my readings were 20 times higher. What this test showed is every time you chew, mercury is released from these toxic fillings. Scary. That test was all the motivation I needed to have them replaced.

The dentist I went to tried to talk me out of removal, noting all my fillings looked good, and there was no need to mess with them. Also, he informed me there was no danger in having mercury in my mouth. I politely asked him to shut up and get on with it. I hope you will have the same conversation with your dentist if he tries to talk you out of removal.

I was bragging to him how I had not been to a dentist in over 25 years because I didn't eat sugar and had an alkaline condition in my mouth as a result of not eating acid forming foods which are a factor in tooth decay. I told him I clean my own teeth, using a stiff bristled toothbrush and an occasional dental pick.

He showed me the error in my ways by documenting my receding gum line. I had damaged my gums through brushing too vigorously. The dental pick was no problem but the hard bristled brush was a problem. I have since stopped brushing hard and use a soft bristled toothbrush. It does seem that my gums have regenerated somewhat. Nowadays I often use my fingers to "brush" my teeth in the shower, thereby avoiding additional wear and tear.

Skin eruptions—as you detoxify your system may well be overwhelmed by the volume of toxins coming out. When you see pimples, blackheads, or even boils start to happen you will know you need to step it up. More hydration. More enemas, more cleansing herbs like Cascara Sagrada. Maybe more rest.

Just tune in and see what your body is asking for. Look for ways to support the cleansing process. Your body is going to start talking to you a lot more now. Listen.

I have stated many times throughout this book that I am in this for the fun. Sometimes though, detoxification is not exactly fun. It is however, what gets you to the fun. You can do this. Stay focused. Some people breeze through the detoxification process. Just keep the faith. You will be ecstatic when you get to the other side of this process. This is just something that has to happen before you can feel amazing. I'm hoping it happens easily for you. Some people want to step up the process. If you're not having a rough time detoxing, then by all means, step it up. The best way to do this is to fast.[14]

Fasting, you will find, is wonderful anytime. It is certainly one reason why poorer countries generally have populations that live longer and with less disease than so-called developed countries. Just try a day at a time and see how you feel. Many people who have done a successful long-term fast have not set out to do so. Oftentimes they just don't feel like eating again so they don't. The amazing "lightness of being" you will experience while fasting will astound you. You need to attain a certain level of cleanness before you get this feeling. Try fasting for one day at first. Maybe start on a Friday night, with the idea of going through Saturday, and then if you feel like it, extend your fast on through Sunday. No need to do it for 40 days and 40 nights like Jesus did. Try it first fasting on juice.

I actually recommend juice fasting for most of your fasting. I have only experimented with water fasting a little. To me the juice fast is so much easier, because you have carbohydrate still coming in, antioxidants in abundance, and something to taste. Perhaps you'd like to try something in between juice and water fasting. A wonderful drink to fast on is water with lemon juice, cayenne, and maple syrup. You can put as much or as little of these into the water as you desire. Often you feel hungry in the beginning of a fast, but soon this sensation ceases. When you do break the fast and start eating, eat lightly, starting with one kind of fruit. Watermelon is an excellent choice for this. Just relax and enjoy the ride. You may find fasting to be the single best thing you could do for your body.

Anytime you use fruit juice, be it as a sports drink or as a fasting staple, you can dilute it with water to lessen the impact the sugar has on you. Some people actually prefer the taste of fruit juice in diluted form.

Pimples or boils appear on the skin when the body is overwhelmed with toxins and the skin is being used as an organ of elimination. If this happens to you don't worry, just step up your efforts at ushering the toxins out of the body. One very common side effect of detoxing is low energy. Don't let this derail you. Many people have had the experience of cleaning up their diet and feeling worse after a short period of feeling better. What's happening is that by not eating the heavy poisonous foods anymore the body has gone into detox mode. You gave it a break by not eating the junk, so now it is cleansing. This can be the end of your healthy diet if you're not careful—and patient.

So many people have told me that when they went on the healthier diet they felt like crap. When they ate their junk, again they felt better because eating it stopped the detox process. When somebody has experienced this, they are not often open to hearing the explanation that they were detoxing, and that all they needed was a little patience and maybe some well-placed enemas or herbal laxatives. All they know is rabbit food = feeling bad, supposed junk food = feeling good. The actual message is; your body is much more toxic than you know. Care must be taken when changing your diet for the better, to keep pace with its need to detox. Help it every step of the way to detox in the ways we have discussed. You will be richly rewarded.

A great way to increase your detoxification of solid waste i.e. poop, is to increase your intake of vitamin C. Every nut milk drink I make I add a heaping teaspoon of vitamin C powder to. This represents about 6000 mg. We always want to poop more. The vitamin C powder actually imparts a little bitterness to your drink. I have gotten used to this, but if you don't want this bitterness in what you are drinking, stir the powder into a small glass of water and drink quickly like a shot, without swirling it around in your mouth. Dramatically increasing your vitamin C levels supports detoxification in many other ways as well. Vitamin C will prove to be the best ally in the detoxing process.

Chemical laxatives work by irritating the walls of the colon, making it want to expel the irritant. You can easily become dependent on them. Some people have found that after a short time taking them they are unable to "go" without this effect. Herbal laxatives like Cascara Sagrada do not irritate the walls of the colon and so don't make you dependent on them. Herbal laxatives, like enemas and colonics, gently "train" the colon to go more easily and frequently. The cleaner you get, the more you will go. Herbs seem not to work so well after taking them for a few days, so it's good to cycle on and off of them and to use different herbs or formulations, Vitamin C doesn't seem to lose any of its laxative effect at all—ever. Here's hoping you make high doses of this most potent of nutrient part of your everyday life.

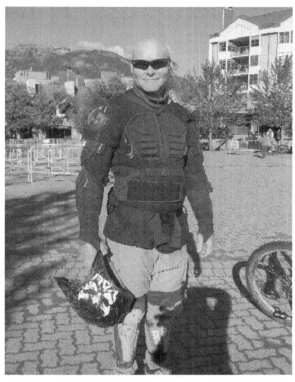

Armored up for first time at Whistler Bike Park downhill

"It is not true that people stop pursuing dreams because they grow old, they grow old because they stop pursuing dreams."

- Gabriel García Márquez

CHAPTER 18
AGEs THAT ARE AGING YOU

N ow, I would like to tell you about a very aptly named factor in aging. It's called advanced glycation end products or AGE's. This process causes wrinkling, cataracts, loss of skin elasticity, loss of vigor in the vital organs and many other symptoms of aging. You can get more information about this process by Googling "advanced glycation end products." This is a newly appreciated cause of aging.[1]

Once again, meat is at the heart of this attack on your heart. If you ate meat raw, it would not be nearly as dangerous as when cooked, especially at high temperatures. Grilling and frying are especially damaging.[2] You can visualize the glycation process by picturing a chicken browning in the oven. This process is actually, what happens in your body. Here's how it works: Your tissues "brown" and thicken due to what has been termed "cross linking."

Cross-linking is known to represent an irreversible modification of protein. Glycation is what causes cataracts. The lens tissue becomes opaque due to thickening and cross-linking. I'm not going to tell you this is irreversible because I have found as long as there is life force in the body, and the daily insults to it stop, the body can be regenerated. However, most experts will tell you this process cannot be reversed and once the tissue is damaged in this way, there is no reversing it. Of course, they don't know about the power of stopping all junk food. Regeneration is not possible if you keep putting the crap in your body, even in small amounts.

Carnosine, one of the amino acids associated with muscle building, has been shown to reduce glycation throughout the body. This is very exciting, the fact that one nutrient can actually stop AGEs from forming, at least to some degree. AGEing is such a big deal that anything that can retard the process has to be viewed as very important indeed. Carnosine has many health benefits too numerous to list here. You may want to educate yourself more fully about this miracle amino. Sounds like some cheap insurance against AGEing to me.[3] I take it already as one of my muscle building aminos.

High blood sugar is another cause of AGE's. "Carbage" is my word for excess carbohydrates and the wrong kind of carbohydrates, which cause blood sugar spikes. This "carbage" is a high risk factor in all aging processes.[4] This puts wheat consumption almost on the same level as meat at causing damage to the body. You will recall nothing spikes your blood sugar like flour products. The simple carbohydrate (pure glucose) in wheat hits your bloodstream like an atom bomb. You could say nothing ages you like a sandwich. As we know, protein and starch eaten together are never properly digested. When you feel the difference of not eating like this, you will never eat another "agewich" again.

You can think of AGE's as the debris that forms and accumulates in the tissues because of these continuing blood sugar spikes and consumption of dead, decaying animal matter. There are two ways that AGE's are formed in your body; endogenous, meaning they are caused by processes inside the body, and exogenous, meaning you eat them directly in food.[5]

It turns out "carbage" is the cause of endogenous AGE formation. Sugar is another example while worse still is high fructose corn syrup (HFCS), fabricated sugar.

You probably know by now, if you have kept up at all with health findings and even the mainstream media, this is not something you want to ingest. Problem is HFCS is in virtually all prepared foods.

The other man made carbohydrate that is so harmful is bread and all wheat products. As we discussed earlier, wheat is particularly adept at spiking blood sugar because it easily becomes pure glucose, needing very little processing. One reason is that bread and flour products have a carbohydrate called amylopectin-A, which is very easily converted into glucose by the enzyme amylase.[6] It is now being appreciated that the wrong kind of carbohydrates are extremely dangerous. Even the good carbohydrates, like fruit juice can spike your blood sugar and cause this inflammatory cascade and increased glycation. There is a time and place for everything though. Time and place control, largely, whether glycation will occur with a given amount of carbohydrates or not. If you are very active and need fuel immediately, glycation does not occur as readily. This is also true of the wrong kind of fats. They are much less harmful if your body is in an active state.

I heard of an experiment where the subject was asked to eat a standard American breakfast containing a large amount of what we would consider the wrong fats. Four hours later, some blood was drawn and run through a centrifuge separating the fat, which rose to the top of the vial and looked like a waxy, oily substance. He was then asked to walk vigorously for two hours that evening. The next day, he ate the same breakfast and was tested again. This time there was much less fat in the blood. What this is showing is when you are active, more of the fat will be made available for use as fuel, and less will be carried by the blood to where it does damage, such as your arteries.[7]

The same is true of carbohydrates. If you need them right now for fuel, carbs will not cause glycation as much.

For many years, I have used fruit juice as my sports drink. It's amazing more athletes haven't discovered this. Fruit juice is the perfect sports drink because you get hydration, antioxidants, and carbohydrates all in one package that needs very little digestion. Add coconut water to fruit juice and you get even more electrolytes in your sports drink. Remember you can always dilute juice to taste if you don't want as much of the sugar it contains.

Riders in the Tour de France are known to eat candy and soft drinks to get quick energy. They are missing the greatest sports drink known to man. Because of their high demand for energy, however, they have far less glycation because of immediately using the energy from the junk food they consumed. Some of them have crappy diets. They work out so often and so hard, they seem to get away with this. Certainly, they don't accumulate fat because they are so active.(being in their 20s and 30s doesn't hurt either) However, as they age, they lose their competitive edge.

We as athletes could be getting better and better as we age. We learn more about our bodies, and how they work in extreme conditions. We get better at our sports, at least the technical aspects, which explains why older athletes can sometimes compete with younger ones. Seems about the time we really connect with the skill part, and learn to pace ourselves more efficiently, the body starts to break down. Again, 40 seems to be the magic number, although the decline happens long before forty for many.

Many athletes are fit but not healthy. I submit this is a result of the crap they eat. Case in point; I read about a coach in Colorado Springs, I can't remember his name, who coached elite bicycle road racers. He went out for a lunchtime ride one day and suffered a massive heart attack, which proved fatal. He was 52. An autopsy showed he had seriously occluded arteries.

199

He was known for his daily ice cream fix. He was so active; he never had to watch what he ate for fear of putting on weight. This proved to be his undoing. He looked and performed great right up to his last day.

I'm finding out if an athlete uses fruit juice as fuel instead of those chemical laden energy gels, and the dreaded Gatorade, which even looks like antifreeze, and doesn't eat junk, he can continue to improve. People often ask me if this or that sports drink is any good. I just say, "Read the ingredients." If you can't pronounce some of the ingredients, you don't want to drink it.

Lately, beet juice has been getting quite a bit of press as an exercise supplement. Probably the ultimate sports drink would be beet juice and celery juice together, especially if you're about to work out in extreme heat. Celery juice, due to its high organic sodium content, helps us cope with intense heat. Experimentation is the key. The more you get to know your body and what it actually thrives on, as opposed to just exists on, the better an athlete you will be.

Now, let's talk about the other way AGEs form in your body. Exogenous AGEs are eaten. Animal products are the culprit. The higher the temperature dead flesh is cooked, the more glycation you get. Cured meats may be worst of all. The higher the temperature and the longer meats are cooked, the richer the AGE content. Fried foods, and anything cooked at high temperatures also contain AGEs. Your potato chips and French fries are anything but "empty" calories. They come loaded with AGEs. Grilled and smoked meats are particularly damaging also.

Blood hemoglobin, which is the part that carries oxygen throughout the body, also becomes glycated. Since blood is renewed every 30 to 60 days, there is a test that will tell you how fast glycation is proceeding in your body. The percentage of hemoglobin molecules in blood that are glycated gives a very good reference for how fast glycation is progressing in the body.[8] Glycation of hemoglobin is also going to decrease your ability to absorb oxygen. This will leave you tired and aging at an accelerated rate.

To sum up, the lesson is; the higher the glucose level in your blood when not needed immediately for energy, and the more meat, and fried food you eat, the faster AGEing will occur.

One more place in the body I might mention as an example of AGEing is the corpus cavernosium or spongeform tissue in the male member. As this tissue becomes glycated, it becomes less spongy. Erection happens when blood flows into the spongiform tissue and is able to be held there. As this tissue glycates, it becomes less able to hold the blood, and therefore, the erection.[9]

Older men often have the symptom of being able to get an erection but not keep it. This is why. Youthful tissue is soft, supple, and flexible. Older tissue is hard (but not in the way you want), inflexible and dense.

There is much continuing research into the cause-and-effect of AGE's. Many health professionals are unaware of these processes. I hope you will educate yourself more about how all this works. I hope especially you will experience these processes slowing down and even reversing in your own body! Remember, if you do what everyone else does, you will age at the accelerated rate that they are currently experiencing. You could say there is a war on. Your body is the battlefield. It is your choice who wins. Are you going to let AGE's have their way with you or are you going to stop waging war on your own body? You have a choice. Knowledge is power. Ignorance is anything but bliss.

Leonardo da Vinci was quoted as saying, "I am a disciple of experience." The quote is sometimes translated, as "I am a disciple of experimentation." To me, they say the same thing. There is no need to take anyone's word for anything, especially since these words change so often, as one-day coffee is bad for you, the next day it's a health food. Give yourself the gift of experience. Give yourself the gift of regeneration. Have the experience of aging in reverse. No one can take this gift away from you. No one will be able to tell you age reversal is not possible. Remember, there is no need to believe or disbelieve anything; experience is all that matters.

Red wine is another substance like coffee and chocolate that used to be thought of as bad for you, now is being looked at as beneficial to the body. Red wine has antioxidants and anthocyanins from the grape juice it used to be. It also has resveratrol, which is certainly a beneficial nutrient. Alcohol though, is something your body will steer you away from when you get clean and healthy. If you stop drinking all alcohol during your detox period, it will go much easier and quicker. If you drink it again after abstaining for about six months you will totally feel how toxic it is.

Your erstwhile experimenter tried drinking wine in 1996. I drink about a glass and a half just to see what would happen. Having only drunk alcohol a few times in the early 70s, and never liking the taste, I choked it down. I never liked the buzz of alcohol. It felt very numbing to me. I especially didn't like the way I felt the next day. I felt nothing after drinking the glass and a half of wine. The next day I slept until well after noon, feeling extremely tired. I got up for a few hours, and went back to bed and slept all the next night. Though the wine never made me nauseous, I felt lethargic for days afterward. Red wine is good for you? I'm not buying it.

I would like to hip you now to another sign of internal aging, which is recently emerging from the scientific literature. It is called lipofuscin. This is a yellow brown deposit of cellular garbage that is deposited throughout the body. It shows up in many ways, and manifests as increased oxidative stress, decreased energy production, and ultimately cell death. On the skin, lipofuscin shows up as 'liver spots'.[10] This is further evidence that aging takes many forms in your body, but the result is largely the same.

Stiffening, darkening, hardening, dehydrating, depleting are all hallmarks of aging. We suffer more and more as we age from all the toxins we ingest. We make less of the hormones and neurotransmitters we need. Lipofuscin and glycation do their dirty work. Muscles atrophy and erections become a fond memory. Understanding these processes can help motivate us to stop them and even to reverse them. Nature has provided us with many helpers.

In the case of erectile dysfunction, I have read about some good herbs; I can't attest to their efficacy, as I haven't experimented with them. Until you reverse your age, you may benefit from yohimbe, damiana, tribulous tredensis, and several others that help with erectile dysfunction. A Google search should turn up many more. There are many herbal formulations to help with ED. Nature has a cure for everything.

Herbs usually have many benefits other than the reason you are taking them. You could call them positive side effects, as opposed to the negative side effects of drugs. Lotsa fun.

Getting back to lipofuscin, a nutrient has emerged as our savior. Creatine. Athletes have been taking creatine for decades to enhance muscle growth and recovery. I have used it for many years myself. Creatine is becoming known for its role in reducing lipofuscin and increasing glucose tolerance. Thereby, mitigating the damage glucose can do through glycation, slowing sarcopenia, and slowing the progression of Alzheimer's, Parkinson's, Huntington's, and Lou Gehrig's diseases. Aging leads to the accumulation of dysfunctional mitochondria, which are the energy factories in each of your cells. Creatine helps keep these energy centers healthy, vibrant, and functioning at a high level. Creatine also enhances the survival and protection of neurons that produce dopamine, one of the 'feel good' neurotransmitters.

Strokes occur because of insufficient blood flow to one or more areas of the brain, often caused by excessive amounts of lipofuscin, as well as arterial plaque. Creatine supplementation goes a long way toward slowing and reversing this process. Creatine has also been shown to help diabetics by increasing the production of the glucose transporter complex called GLUT-4. GLUT-4 shuttles sugar molecules from the blood into cells and on to the mitochondria, where instead of being stored as fat, it can be used as energy. Animal experiments have shown a 9% increase in lifespan by Creatine supplementation alone. This is not as impressive as the 50% increase animal experiments have demonstrated for CR, or calorie restriction, but pretty cool nonetheless.

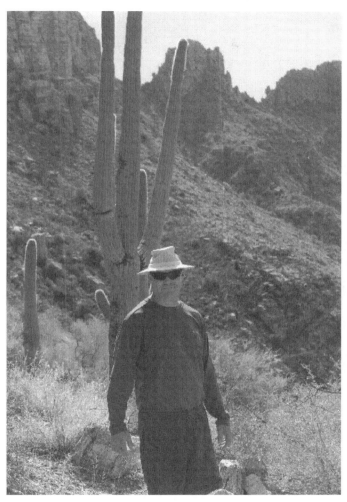

Hiking Sabino Canyon Trail, Tucson

"The art of medicine consists of amusing the patient while nature cures the disease."

                                                        - Voltaire

CHAPTER 19
SUPER FOODS & SUPPLEMENTS

R aw organic vegetables would have to be considered the ultimate super foods. For centuries, humankind has known that vegetables and fruits were health foods. Now we know why. It's not just about the vitamins and minerals they contain. They also fortify your body with antioxidants and phytonutrients.

Mushrooms are one of the few foods that naturally have vitamin D. Mushrooms; you will find can be used to replace meat in dishes. We are even seeing Portobello mushrooms being used in sandwiches in place of the meat in restaurants and delis. Mushrooms of all kinds add many interesting flavors to anything. Mushrooms have many health benefits, as well as tastes and textures.

Onions are foods we want to experiment with, and use in abundance. They share with garlic a substance called alicin, which has been known to cure cancer in enough concentration. There are whole books written on the wonders of this miracle substance. With so many different kinds of onions available, the culinary possibilities are endless. Try different ones, and consume them as raw as possible. There is variety called Vidalia, after the Georgia town where they are grown, that are sweet enough to juice and drink straight. I hope you experiment with onions, and grow to love them.

Nuts and seeds must be added to our list of super foods. Nuts actually are seeds. As such, they contain enough life force to grow a tree. They are extremely nutrient dense. The EFA's so lacking in most people's diets, are very well represented in any nut or seed. EFA's (essential fatty acids) will keep your skin soft and supple. The skin of your internal organs will also be kept supple and functional with the inclusion of more EFA's in your diet. The brain also thrives on the right kind of fats. No doubt, EFA's help you preserve brain function as you age. Walnuts in particular are known as the ultimate brain food. Brazil nuts are rich in selenium, which is a vitally important nutrient very poorly supplied by most people's diets. This list could go on and on, but I'll leave it there. Further research and experimentation is an adventure that awaits you.

Now, I'll tell you about one of the most underappreciated and cheapest to supplement nutrients out there. It's known as Vitamin D, but in the body, it acts more like a hormone. It is involved in too many body processes to list here. New research shows Vitamin D to have a role in more and more body systems all the time.[1]

It was thought, until recently, we could get all the Vitamin D we needed from minimal sunlight exposure, as the body synthesizes it from sunlight exposure to the skin. Now, Vitamin D is being shown to be severely depleted and deficient in most people. People with dark skin get less than people with lighter skin as dark pigmented skin blocks more sunlight absorption. In fact, Vitamin D is the reason we have the different human races. If you'll allow me to digress for a moment.

Modern humans evolved in Africa only about 200,000 years ago. We moved out of Africa at a very slow rate starting only about 40,000 years ago. This has all been proven scientifically through DNA research.[2] As we moved north, the skin had to lighten to absorb the available Vitamin D. Climates that are more northern had less available sunlight and we had to cover ourselves to stay warm. The humans that moved the furthest north developed the lightest skin. Therefore, up until about 20,000 to 30,000 years ago, when we reached northern Europe, and probably contributed to the demise of our cousins, the Neanderthals, all modern humans were black. You can easily grasp the social significance of this.

I laugh when I hear white people who don't like blacks but like sports. If they like basketball or football, most of the players are black. In addition, I hope they don't like rock 'n roll, because black people invented that. It was called the Blues, and it came directly from African rhythms, brought here by slaves. Ray Manzerik, the keyboard player for the Doors, who died in 2013, was quoted as saying, "Without black people, we would all be dancing the Minuet."

If this nutrient single-handedly caused the races to occur, it has to be important. Most health seekers know by now that without sufficient Vitamin D and magnesium; calcium, regardless of type, will not be properly absorbed by the body. I hope you educate yourself more about Vitamin D and its many roles throughout the body. Vitamin D, like NAC, is very inexpensive to supplement. There is no reason not to have enough in your body. Vitamin D3 is the preferred type. It must be taken with some kind of dietary fat. I hope that you are getting plenty of the beneficial fats we talked about earlier. CoQ10 also needs to be taken with some type of fat.

I have another fancy word for you: immunosenescence. This is a slowing down of your body's manufacture of antibodies, lymphocytes, and killer B cells. Along with the slowing down of the body's production of glutathione, we start to manufacture less of the protective 'killer' cells that attack microbes and potential cancer cells. You could say, we lose vitality and vigor in our immune function. When the immune system is out of balance in this way, we not only lose the ability to counteract threats but also the strict control of inflammation goes out the window. Inflammation gone out of control is at the heart of virtually all disease systems.

This is newly recognized stuff. Inflammation is now emerging as the root cause of all disease at the cellular level. Here again, nature has provided us with something to halt and reverse immunosenescence.[3]

It's called Rishi mushroom. You can buy it in supplement form. Rishi is very easy to add to your supplement protocol. It has been shown to single-handedly eradicate cancer cells, even after they become full-blown cancers. If you opt for chemotherapy, Rishi will enhance it, making chemo work better. However, many people who try Rishi first don't opt for chemotherapy at all.

Rishi also promotes dendritic cells and macrophages, which allow you to react to threats such as cells mutating out-of-control and invading pathogens. Rishi triggers growth and development of bone marrow where most immune cells are born.

Bone marrow lost to chemotherapy has been regenerated by the use of Rishi supplementation. It stimulates production and function of all natural killer cells. It suppresses inflammatory cytokines produced during chronic inflammation. Rishi has also been shown to help with asthma and allergic response.

We always have cells that start to mutate in weird ways. In other words, we always have cancer cells. Whether these cells are allowed to grow and proliferate is a question of how well your immune system is able to kill them off. Rishi increases immunosurveillance, the body's ability to track and identify cancer cells, targeting them for destruction before they become dangerous.

One way Rishi is able to kill cancer cells even if they have become solid tumors is to choke off their blood supply. The polysaccharides in Rishi fight new blood vessel development in solid tumors, which halts their rapid growth, and begins to kill them off. Rishi also helps you to fight off both bacterial and viral infections. Antibiotics, as we know, are only effective against bacteria. Pretty cool huh?

Like with chemotherapy, Rishi can work alongside antibiotics, enhancing their efficacy. Rishi has also been shown especially effective against viruses of the herpes family, which include chickenpox and shingles. My neighbor, who is up in years, had a bad case of shingles on one side of his face, which turned into full-blown neuralgia. I wish I had known about Rishi. Of course, he may or may not have been interested. People of that age may not be inclined to try treatments their doctor has not recommended. Certainly if he asked his doctor about Rishi, he would not have been encouraged to try it. Ah well, we can only do what our conditioning allows us to do.

I have also read that Rishi helps prevent herpes outbreaks. Many people who have herpes, of which there are many, take a drug called Valtrex to keep outbreaks from happening. I've read that as much as 70% of the population in America has the herpes simplex two virus. Many people do not know they carry herpes, so continue to spread it. If Rishi can stop the cold sore like pimples that characterize herpes from occurring, maybe you can cure herpes completely. It wouldn't surprise me.

Rishi has been shown in animal studies to increase longevity by 10%. As you know from listening to my narrative, longevity doesn't matter much to me. I'm all about feeling good NOW. I am interested in feeling and performing better and better as I age. Now at almost 60, I feel better than I have ever felt in my whole life.

Cancers rarely happen in younger people, yet as we age, our risk for cancer grows with every passing year. Why is this? As we age, our immune systems experience greater and greater rates of senescence. As we lose immune function, we become more and more at risk for diseases of all kinds. Rishi helps us maintain immune function deep into old age. There is one more plant helper I would like to tell you about that also helps us maintain our immune systems, and even regenerate failing ones. It is a flower that as long been used in traditional Chinese medicine. It is called Cistanche.

Cistanche primarily helps to strengthen your adaptive immune system. Rishi helps mainly with your innate immune system. Your innate immune system is your body's first line of defense against invaders. It is the part that is activated by vaccinations. The innate immune system "learns" which pathogens are dangerous, and has tailored itself to targeting those it has faced in the past. The adaptive immune system stands ready to hunt down and destroy pathogens the immune system has not faced before. As we age the adaptive immune system, once so healthy and vigorous in our youth, begins to slow down.

T cells can be considered the "brains" of the immune system. They are also known as killer cells. There are two basic types adaptive or "naïve", and innate or "memory" T cells. Naïve T cells once they have responded to a threat become memory cells. Memory T cells are programed to respond to a specific threat that has previously been faced by the body. New threats must be handled by naïve T cells. As we age, we build up a greater inventory of memory T cells. We may actually be better able to respond to threats we have faced before then a younger person. In creating these memory cells however, naïve T cells are depleted.

This depletion of naïve T cells is the reason older people do not respond to new threats to the body as well as younger people. New threats are constantly emerging, like new strains of the flu and cancer cells that take new forms and trigger the growth of new carcinogens. This may be the main reason older people are more susceptible to cancers and viruses of all types.

Cistanche helps the body create new naïve T cells. To my knowledge, nothing else does this. This is a very inexpensive supplement. The extract form is available from Life Extension Foundation for about $10 a bottle. Rishi is also available from them at a low price. Supplementing with these two inexpensive miracle plants could enhance your immune system and preserve your ability to fight off invaders and kill cancer cells. Cistanche has not been widely available, to my knowledge, until recently. I just ordered some after reading about it. Why not? I have been taking Rishi for years. Now I have something else to bolster my immune system.

I want to tell you about another proven cancer cure. It comes from the crocus flower. Saffron consists of the dried dark red or yellow stigmas of the flower crocus sativaus. The active ingredients are called crocin, crocetin, and safranal. You can avail yourself of the healing properties of saffron by consuming the spice or by taking it in supplement form. LEF has a formulation called "Optimized Saffron". Saffron has been proven to prevent carcinogenesis, which means it stops tumors from forming. A study was done where animals were orally treated with saffron prior to administration of a powerful chemical carcinogen. Tumor formation was completely prevented, proving saffron's ability to prevent cancer. A quote from LEF magazine, March 2015: "Saffron extracts and specific components have also been shown to potently prevent DNA damage caused by free radicals, radiation, and inflammation, thereby reducing the risk of new cancer formation." Additionally, "Once a cell has been triggered to become malignant it then proliferates, or reproduces rapidly and without normal controls, to produce a developing tumor. Studies show that saffron is able to suppress—and in some cases reverse– the proliferation of certain human cancer cells in culture. For example, one compelling study found that cancer cells that were treated with either saffron extract– or its major component, crocin– displayed sharp and significant reductions in proliferation, to as low as 2.8% of the rate seen in untreated cells. A similar reduction in proliferation was demonstrated in lung cancer and breast cancer as well."

Saffron also fights cancer by restoring cell's responsiveness to apoptosis, or programmed cell death. Cancer cells typically lose their responsiveness to the apoptosis signal, effectively becoming "immortal" and hence deadly. A further quote: "if a cancer cell survives attempts to quash it by blocking proliferation or apoptosis, it may go on to produce specialized molecules that help it degrade the protein matrix between healthy cells, allowing it to invade otherwise healthy tissue. This is how cancer spreads locally, and is also a major mechanism in metastasis, the spread of malignant cells throughout the body." Saffron blocks this action and blocks the introduction of new blood vessel growth that feeds the malignancy. This growth is called angiogenesis. "Recent studies support the use of saffron extracts in reducing levels of a vital signaling molecule called vascular endothelial growth factor, which markedly reduces new blood vessel formation in the tumor mass."

Another use of Saffron is to prevent and cure metabolic syndrome, which as we know is a combination of obesity, insulin resistance, high blood sugar, inflammation, lipid abnormalities, and hypertension, and is a major risk factor for cardiovascular disease. Anything that can help us to cure metabolic syndrome is in itself a godsend.

If that was not enough reason to take it, there is also the fact that it has been proven to protect your heart. We have seen in earlier chapters how the wrong kind of calcium causes artery occlusion. To quote LEF again: "In a mechanism similar to the common calcium channel blocking drugs, saffron inhibits the inflow of calcium into smooth muscle cells and artery walls and in heart muscle tissue, a process known to constrict arteries and raise blood pressure."

Saffron also protects your brain. Its effect on oxidation, inflammation, and glucose damage show it to be a powerful neuroprotective agent against both neurodegenerative disease and mood disorders such as depression, which affects upwards of one-fifth of the US population. It has been shown to greatly help in the prevention and reversal of neurodegenerative diseases like Alzheimer's and dementia. Pretty impressive for a supplement that costs $24 for 60 capsules, and you only need to take two a day.

Now, I'm very excited to share with you a proven cure for Alzheimer's (dementia) and Parkinson's. This should have been front-page news when it was shown to prevent and reverse these supposedly inevitable symptoms of ageing. In this country, natural cures get very little press. Vinpocetine has been used since the 70s in Europe and Japan to treat not only the aforementioned diseases, but circulatory issues and hearing problems as well.

It is an established fact now that cognitive and neurodegenerative disease is caused by the same thing as cardiovascular disease—occluded arteries and decreased blood flow. In other words, cognitive impairment is caused by cardiovascular issues. We all know someone with Alzheimer's or Parkinson's. Millions of Americans are affected, and the number is going up fast as the "baby boomers" hit their later years. Vinpocetine, a derivative of the Periwinkle plant directly treats hypo perfusion (decreased blood flow).

To quote an LEF magazine article on the subject: "Total cerebral blood flow is 20% lower in Alzheimer's disease patients than in those without dementia. Studies have shown that constant low blood flow to the brain is often a marker for whether or not someone will develop Alzheimer's." What is the root cause of this decrease in blood flow? Saturated (animal) fat and the resultant high triglycerides, and LDL cholesterol, of course. How can we restore blood flow to the brain? Stop eating animal products and take Vinpocetine. Simple. So many people live in fear of Alzheimer's disease – this horrible thief of your personality. Our bodies degenerating as we age is scary enough, but losing our minds? What could be worse than that?

Another LEF quote: "Research demonstrates that Vinpocetine exerts anti-atherogenic effects on blood vessels and enhances brain blood flow. These brain-protective effects are a result of a host of mechanisms induced by Vinpocetine. Vinpocetine directly relaxes vascular smooth muscle, making it an extremely powerful vasodilator." "Vinpocetine exerts viscosity lowering effects on blood and plasma. It also decreases platelet and red blood cell aggregation, boosts red blood cell membrane flexibility, and exhibits clinically substantiated anti-ischemic activity." So now, we are seeing how strokes caused by blood clots or decreased blood flow to one or more areas of the brain can be potentially eradicated by supplementation with Vinpocetine.

Vinpocetine has been used successfully to enhance memory, and even reverse memory loss due to old age. New research is showing, as I shared with you earlier, the brain can be regenerated to a degree science had deemed impossible until recently. The old myth that there was nothing we could do about brain atrophy (shrinkage), memory loss, and cognitive decline, is being replaced with a new appreciation for the brain's ability to adapt and respond to positive changes in lifestyle. When we begin to work with instead of against our bodies and our brains, we can reverse all symptoms of aging.

Tinnitus, the constant ringing in the ears some people experience due to age, or to hearing damage from exposure to loud noise, especially over long periods, is said to be helped by Vinpocetine. I have mild tinnitus myself, from many years of playing loud music in small rooms before I discovered the blessing of earplugs. After reading about how Vinpocetine helps with tinnitus, I decided to order some. To my delight, I found this an extremely inexpensive supplement. Who knows? The fact that it helps with vascular issues may mean it will increase athletic performance as well. I guess I'm about to find out.

CoQ10 and circumin have been used successfully to slow the progression of Parkinson's disease. There is no drug cure for Parkinson's or Alzheimer's. All drugs can do in the case of Parkinson's is possibly decrease the shaking and other symptoms, as the disease gets worse and worse. In Vinpocetine, we may now actually have a cure for this incredibly debilitating disease! This nutraceutical (a drug derived from a plant) holds the key. It seems to reverse the ravages of old age on our brains. This inexpensive supplement will be part of my supplement protocol for the rest of my life. Better safe than sorry. Nothing could be worse than shaking uncontrollably (Parkinson's), or losing memory and brain function (Alzheimer's) in our later years. Now we know this doesn't have to happen, and indeed won't happen, if we stop consuming the substances that cause decreased blood flow to the brain, and start supplementing with a proven brain protector and vascular system enhancer. It's your call.

As I shared with you before, I have been an athlete all my life. I have been cleansing my internal body since I was 21. The way my physical body feels now defies description. You will have this feeling too. Advancing years will bring you an advancing high! This is the buzz that never ends. Well, certainly, the physical part will end, but I don't care. Right now is all we will ever have. This moment is the playing field the game of life is played on. If you are not enjoying this moment, if you are not feeling good now, you have the keys in your hand to change it up. Don't let compulsion, addiction, and preconceived notions rob you of this opportunity.

I have talked a bit about how cancers form and what you can do to stop them from forming, and if formed, to stop them from proliferating. Don't let anyone tell you there is no cure for cancer. Maitake mushrooms, as well as Rishi, are showing themselves to be cancer cures. I read an account where Maitake was used by a man awaiting removal of his stomach, diagnosed as cancerous. After using the Maitake, his appointment day arrived and the stomach was removed. A subsequent biopsy of the removed stomach showed the cancer was gone. Too bad, they didn't check the stomach before removal.[4]

The problem is you don't hear about these alternative cures in the mainstream media. There seems to be some major censorship going on. Could it be that cancer has become an industry, and that government and the media are protecting the industry? There's a doctor in Texas who has developed his own cure for cancer, from horse urine no less, and has faced incredible obstacles. He has been persecuted by the FDA and the state of Texas because he has a cure that works. He has spent millions defending himself with much of the money donated by his patients who were cured of terminal cancer. His name is Dr. Burzynski.[5] If you search his name, you will be able to watch his documentary that takes you through this story. It is truly fascinating, and very enlightening as to what is going on.

We must educate ourselves not just about what is and isn't good for us, but about how our world and our government works. I find delving into mysteries both spiritual and natural to be a source of continuing wonderment and joy. It has been rewarding also to do research into the stories behind the story, if you know what I mean. If we delve deeper without fear, just for our own edification, it can be a lot of fun. I'm the type of person who wants to know the truth. Whether it's good news or bad news, I want to know what's up.

I would like to share a few more supplements and super foods with you. It's hard to know where to start, and especially where to end, as there are so many supplements I have used or read about. I hope you will learn more and more about all the wonderful herbs, vitamins, minerals, cofactors, and amino acids available to help you regain your youth and even feel better than you did in your youth. I recommend the Life Extension Foundation and their fantastic magazine that comes out monthly. The magazine is a source of cutting-edge new research and development in the field of longevity and youth reclaiming. Anyway, here is the short list of a few supplements and super foods that are very dear to my heart– and to the rest of my body as well.

Seaweed is a form of algae, which is a very simple plant. Algae, like mushrooms are unique classes of plants with many medicinal properties.[6] Astaxanthin is a red pigment in algae that gives salmon its red color, one reason salmon is touted as such a health food. You can take Astaxanthin directly in supplement form and save yourself from ingesting mercury and other toxins; you would receive if you ate the salmon. It has been shown to protect from sunburn and skin damage. It has even been called an internal sunscreen. Like any of these supplements, I'm telling you about, you can learn much more through a Google search, and asking knowledgeable health professionals and health food store employees about whatever supplement interests you.

Blue-green algae and Spirolina are fairly well known for their long list of health benefits. Spirolina, with its rich dark green color, is packed with chlorophyll. Chlorella is another form of algae that is known for its high chlorophyll content.[7] The molecular structure of chlorophyll, I have read, is one molecule different from hemoglobin, the part of your blood that transports oxygen. This is one reason why green foods are so healing and healthy for us.

There are many types of seaweeds, all with amazing health benefits. Thyroid issues are epidemic in this country, many of them undiagnosed. Iodine is the nutrient the thyroid needs most for proper function. Iodine is extremely rare in the diets of developed countries, which is why it was added to table salt in the 50s. Before that time, thyroid enlargement was common. The thyroid enlarges in an effort to do its many jobs throughout the body when it is not given enough iodine to function properly. This growth can get so extreme as to manifest itself as a goiter. Putting iodine in table salt has largely eradicated goiters. However, since iodine is not stable in table salt, and more savvy health-conscious people avoid salt, most people do not get anywhere near enough. This is one of the main causes of low thyroid function or Hypothyroidism. Also known as underactive thyroid, you may well have it even if you are asymptomatic.[8]

Oddly enough, the thyroid can also be overactive. This is called hyperthyroidism. I met a woman who had this in the form of Grave's disease. I jokingly said, "That sounds serious". I said, "They really should call that something else". She was not amused as this disease lessened her quality of life quite a bit. The medication she was on was not working. I suggested eating lots of seaweed and getting not only iodine, but also lots of readily absorbable calcium and chlorophyll, as well as trace minerals, in the bargain. She replied, "I don't like seaweed." I restrained my laughter and said, "Okay let me get this straight, you've got a disease robbing you of your quality of life, but you won't try something that has been known to help, especially if the drug isn't working?" As far as I know, she never did try it.

Another great sea vegetable is called dulse. It is a purple seaweed with a very mild flavor, and adds a bit of saltiness, if you like that, to any dish or drink. You can get dulse in leaf form or granulated. The granulated form can be sprinkled on salads, soups, or whatever you're making. This stuff packs some serious nutrition. Not only is iodine present, but also many trace minerals that are in extremely short supply, even in the best diet. I highly recommend you give up salt, even the fancy natural salts, like Himalayan sea salt, and Celtic Sea salt in favor of dulse that can add saltiness to a dish. Sure, these salts are better than the more commercial brands, which are bleached, but salt is the enemy of cellular water.

Contrary to popular belief, we do not need salt. What we do need is organic sodium. Sodium has to be balanced by potassium. Most people's sodium/potassium balance is way off, because they consume salt. Potassium is found in vegetables, which are in short supply in most diets. Organic sodium is extremely abundant in celery. Celery juice is one of the greatest things to consume before you work out or do anything else in the heat.

We can learn to like whatever we want to learn to like. There is no one deciding you don't like it but you. There are also many different varieties of seaweed for experimentation. Getting a little bit off the subject of seaweed for second, let me share with you my experience at learning to like something. In 1976, I read about wheatgrass. Wheatgrass was not exactly mainstream at that time. Now, most health seekers have at least heard of it. Back then, you couldn't walk into a juice bar or a

Whole Foods and get a shot of wheatgrass. You had to grow your own. After reading about this miraculous health food, I decided to do just that. There was only one juicer available that would juice wheatgrass. It was a small cast-iron hand crank model. I grew the grass, got the juicer, and prepared for my first taste of this wondrous substance.

To say I didn't like the wheatgrass juice would be a severe understatement. I've heard people say they loved it the first time they tasted it and continue to love it. For whatever reason, I wasn't feeling it. I decided though, I wanted to avail myself of the benefits of this superfood. Therefore, I resolved to like it. I started mixing it with carrot juice, which helped quite a bit. Subsequently, I had my first experience with changing the thought around taste, and thereby, changing the reality. Within a very short time, I loved wheatgrass and still do. My motto for many years after that was "you decide". Our tastes can change any time we want them to. You are the master of your sense of taste. Period. It's all part of reclaiming our free will. It's a lot of fun to connect with your unlimited power to create your reality.

You will also have the opposite experience, where you lose the taste for food you used to love. As you eat more and more of the good stuff, your desire for the bad stuff falls away. This is the grace. This is what makes it easy to make decisions and stick to them. All we have to do is focus on what we want, and what we don't want drops out of the picture. Hallelujah.

Okay, back to seaweed. Okinawa, an island off Japan has some of the longest-lived and healthiest people on the planet. It is actually number one on the chart of the longest-lived people in the world. Their longevity doesn't interest me as much as their incredible, by Western standards, lack of disease. Cancer and heart disease were virtually unknown until the Japanese started eating Western diets. Soy is often credited as the reason.

221

The fact is the Japanese eat very little soy. The soy they do eat is mostly in the form of natto and tempeh, which are used as condiments. These are both fermented soy products.

One huge reason for their longevity and lack of disease is their consumption of seaweed. Certainly, their close family ties and close ties to the land and sea play a role as well. New research has uncovered a component in seaweed that may very well explain their longevity. It is called fuccoidan and is present in all seaweeds, but especially the brown variety.[9] There are so many minerals in seaweed that are virtually unavailable anywhere else. You simply have to like seaweed! Nori is the variety pressed into sheets and used to make sushi. Kombu is a variety where the leaves are very thick and robust. Kombu is often soaked and used as a substitute for pasta in raw dishes like lasagna. There are many others to play around with in recipes. Time for some experimentation.

We were talking about immunoscenessence earlier. You'll recall, it is the blanket term for the slowdown of the immune system that occurs with aging. Another supplement helping greatly to prevent this process is Zinc. Zinc is another mineral in short supply in the diets of most people. It is also a precursor, or building block of testosterone, along with selenium, Maca, and ginger. Instead of rubbing on testosterone cream, which will slow down your body's natural manufacture of testosterone, you can up your intake of these minerals and herbs, and reap all their other benefits as well. Give your body the raw materials to make its own testosterone.

Zinc is also known as a pro-sexual nutrient, meaning it increases sex drive, stamina, and desire. It is a very inexpensive mineral to add to your supplement regimen and is found in abundance in pumpkin seeds, which are super foods in their own right. Zinc is known to reduce the risk of infection as well as decrease oxidative inflammatory markers. In one experiment, animals were given a carcinogen, which caused tumors. The group given Zinc experienced 50% less tumor growth.[10]

Zinc has long been known as a great supplement to take during cold and flu season. If you do get a cold, it will shorten the duration and lessen the severity. Zinc also helps in normalizing your metabolism after it has been ravaged by metabolic syndrome. The list could go on and on.

There are probably entire books written about zinc alone. It's right up there with Vitamin C, as a "do all" medicine chest in a capsule. It even helps you avoid macular degeneration, which is a leading cause of blindness and eyesight erosion in the elderly. Neurological disorders, like Parkinson's, have also been helped by Zinc supplementation. It's even been said that Immunoessence is caused by zinc deficiency. It isn't clear if Zinc deficiency is the single-handed cause but the potential connection demonstrates just how important Zinc is to our body.

Here's another herb I particularly like, and one of the few I can actually feel working. It's somewhat new to this country, coming from Russia. It is called Rhodiola. Like all supplements, the extract version is the strongest. Rhodiola helps with energy production, especially stamina.[11] I like to take it before my long bicycle rides. Rhodiola seems to help me concentrate better, which when you're flying downhill on a mountain bike, is a good thing. It has many benefits. I'm trying to keep this little discourse short because you can find more information on supplements and herbs from so many other sources. I'm trying to give you stuff in this book you can't find anywhere else.

Hawthorn is another herb I use to fuel my rides. It's known mostly for its heart and cardiovascular system improvements. Like Rhodiola, you can feel the benefit, almost immediately.[12]

I can't help but comment on the idea of taking low-dose aspirin to help your cardiovascular system. The idea is aspirin thins your blood.[13] Thickening of the blood can cause clotting, leading to phlebitis or stroke. I had vascular surgery in 2004 due to a severely shattered left femur, which tore up a bunch of veins and arteries. The doctor wanted to put me on Coumadin, a blood thinning medication, which has since been shown to have many severe side effects. Instead, I pulled out an herb book and researched which herbs would do the same thing. I found Butchers Broom and Horse Chestnut listed, and began to take them. No complications from the surgery and no side effects from the drugs! If anybody advises you to take aspirin as a preventative to thin your blood, now you know you have alternatives. People taking low-dose aspirin as a preventative, have often paid the price of internal bleeding, leaky gut, and a host of other side effects. Leaky gut has recently been shown to be a course of systemic inflammation. I could go on about the side effects of aspirin, but I'll stop there.

CoQ10 is probably the most important supplement you can take to protect your heart and cardiovascular system. It is also involved in energy production and a long list of other body functions. CoQ10 is also known as Ubiquinol because it is ubiquitous throughout the body. In other words, it's everywhere, helping virtually every function your body performs. Like so many hormones and cofactors, your body makes less CoQ10 as you age which can result in severe depletion.

Cholesterol lowering drugs (statins), as I discussed before, do not stop or even slow down your absorption of cholesterol from food, they block your body's ability to make not only the "bad" LDL, but also the "good" HDL. They also block the manufacture of CoQ10, testosterone, serotonin and other beneficial cofactors and hormones, as these are made along the same pathways.[14]

CoQ10 is getting some notoriety these days as a treatment for Parkinson's disease. CoQ10 can halt the progression, or at least slow Parkinson's down in many cases. There is no cure for Parkinson's disease in the form of drugs. All drugs can do is hope to alleviate the symptoms at this point. Ubiquinol offers hope for real cure. Couple CoQ10 with creatine, zinc, and curcumin, while cleaning up your diet and you might actually have a chance at curing this disease.

Now, let's talk about curcumin.[15] Curcumin is the active ingredient in turmeric. It has been found to not only help with Parkinson's, but also joint issues, arthritis and even depression. Clinical trials have shown that Curcumin can work quite well to help symptoms of depression. Team it up with SAM-e, and you could free yourself from depression forever.

Turmeric is a root in the ginger family. Like ginger, it is cardioprotective. More and more benefits of these two wonder roots are becoming known virtually every day. Ginger is especially useful for stomach upset. Just taking a couple of capsules is often enough to get rid of nausea, and help your hangover. If a couple of capsules don't do the trick, take more. Take as many capsules as you need. Unlike drugs, you can't overdose on herbs, except maybe ephedra.

Ephedra is an herb I like to use on my bike rides. You can definitely feel this one. Sometimes, it's hard to sleep the night after a ride if I take too much. Ephedra gives you a hell of a lift though. It is the only herb I've ever noticed an effect from taking too much.[16]

I've experimented with many different herbs over the years. One herb that has worked very well for clients and friends is White Willow Bark. The original aspirin was a synthesized version of the active ingredient in White Willow

Bark. This active ingredient is called salicylic acid.[17] You can get its pain relieving benefits without taking a drug with associated side effects. It's great for headaches. I once offered some to a woman who used to take over the counter pain medications for frequent headaches. When I offered White Willow Bark, she informed me that an herb could never be strong enough to deal with her headache. I told her to just try it and if two capsules don't work to take four. Two capsules actually did the trick for her. She was mind blown. I guarantee she'll never put herbs down again. I guess the media has helped engender the notion that herbs cannot possibly have the same strong curative effect as drugs. I guess I can't blame her for being skeptical. She's not skeptical now.

Speaking of the curative effect of drugs, their real value is in symptom relief. Treating disease with drugs has been called "crisis management". In crisis management, we want to stop the symptoms before they become life threatening. This approach works very well with trauma from accidents. It doesn't work as well in treating disease systems because it only addresses the symptoms of a disease. These symptoms, like high blood pressure, sometimes need to be treated immediately. The problem is that symptom management does little or nothing to heal the underlying issue. True healing is achieved by removing the cause of disease, not by alleviating its symptoms.

DHEA is a hormone your body makes, but here again, as you age, you make less of it. It is involved in many body functions, and is a good hormone to supplement.[18] Restoring DHEA to youthful levels has many age reversing benefits. It has restored sexual function to more than a few men. DHEA hormone production declines quite severely, up to 80 to 90%, in people over 70. This is a huge deal. Think of all those people in nursing homes being fed all that horrible food, not given any supplements, minimal or no exercise, and being left to waste away. Don't let this happen to you. Take matters into your own hands NOW.

I feel like I'm getting a little carried away with this list, but it's hard to stop. One of the most potent nutrients out there has to be Vitamin E. It is a very powerful antioxidant and protects your body from environmental pollution of all kinds. Vitamin E helps absorb oxygen. When athletes exert themselves in the heat, free radicals can be produced. Vitamin E slows this process. The list of its benefits could fill a book and probably have.

Lots of new research has been done on Vitamin E lately. We have always focused on one type of Vitamin E, called d-alpha tocopheral. At my local health food store, this type is still the only form of vitamin E to be found. It comes in a softgel capsule and is very useful topically for cuts and especially burns. Vitamin E can heal the wound in a fraction of the time it would take without application. It is excellent to use around your eyes to soften and prevent wrinkles. Vitamin E can also act as a sunscreen, and is the best thing you could put on a sunburn. I've had my share, trust me. I'm being more careful these days, but when I get a sunburn, I head straight to the Vitamin E.

New research is focusing on the other two types of tocopherols, and the three types of tocotrenals. These make up what's called "full spectrum" Vitamin E.[19] Research is now showing you need all six, and supplementing with only one of the six may deplete the others, which are in short supply in most people's diets anyway. The d-alpha type is still useful for topical applications, but more enlightened health writers are advising against taking just d-alpha. Most health food stores still do not stock full spectrum Vitamin E. A full-spectrum vitamin E is usually a dry tablet. It's a little expensive, but definitely worth the price. Life Extension Foundation has a good one.[20]

There is an even better way to get your full-spectrum vitamin E and a host of antioxidants and essential fatty acids as well. Red palm oil. This oil is a super food to end all super foods. All the many benefits of olive oil make it an oil you should continue to use. However, you never want to cook with olive oil, as it has a very low "flash point," meaning its molecular structure is altered by heat, turning it from a healthy oil to an unhealthy one. Coconut oil and red palm oil are much better to cook with because they have very high flashpoints.

Red palm oil used to be hard to come by and expensive, but now my local farmers market has it for $12 a gallon. It is a bargain even at the $25 a quart I used to pay. Nothing provides you with full-spectrum vitamin E like this stuff. Red Palm oil is one of few foods to give you a complete Vitamin E profile. It actually tastes good too.[21] Nuts and seeds are also good sources of full spectrum Vitamin E.

I use coconut oil as a moisturizer every day. It's good for cooking and is full of essential fatty acids. It is said Coconut oil and palm oil are the only saturated fats in the vegetable kingdom. This was thought not to matter. As I shared in an earlier chapter, Red palm oil may be the reason my LDL number is not in the optimal range. This bears further research. I'm on it.

Coconut oil is a wonderful sexual lubricant as well. As I write this, I am reminded of something I read which was a quote from George Burn's book entitled "How to live to be 100". He relates a story of getting a check-up from his doctor at age 80. His doctor, remarking on his good health asked him, "So Mr. Burns, you seem in very good health, tell me when your sex life ended?" George replied, "About 3 o'clock this morning." George did live to be 100 and six months.

I guess I'll conclude my list of favorite supplements. I have by no means covered all the supplements I take. I don't take many supplements on a daily basis because some are stored in the body fairly well. Though Vitamin D is a fat-soluble vitamin, it gets flushed out of the body quickly. Most of the fat-soluble vitamins like Vitamin E are stored more readily. The water-soluble vitamins, which include Vitamin C and all the B vitamins are not stored at all, and are destroyed by heat. Therefore, all cooked food is going to have little or no water-soluble vitamins. The less you can cook your food, the better. Of course, you've heard this statement before.

Lightly steaming or even better lightly sautéing with red palm oil and water at a low heat is one of the best ways to cook vegetables. Get the pan hot enough to start sizzling a bit on the bottom, stir the veggies around for a few minutes, and remove from heat and cover, letting the vegetables sit and steam. This process is a good way to cook your vegetables. As you remove from the heat, you can add spices and herbs, letting the vegetables sit and absorb the spices. This is one way to sauté' with minimal cooking. You always want your vegetables to be crunchy. You can also make a blender drink out of vegetables or put them through a food processor for better absorption of nutrients with minimal chewing. Again, experimentation is the key. Use your imagination, and you will find many ways to cook and prepare food. Who knows? Maybe you'll even write a cookbook someday.

To wrap up the rap on supplements, I ask you to keep educating yourself. So many supplements are beneficial. I mentioned the Life Extension Foundation earlier, but neglected to mention they are a great source for supplements. LEF has a discount for buying multiple bottles. And the quality always seems to be quite high. They also have a so-called "super sale" around the first of the year with deep discounts, which is a great time to stock up.

Vitamin B12 is abundant in algae and yeast. Brewer's yeast and nutritional yeast make wonderful additions to salads, soups and other dishes, and are packed with B vitamins. Just be sure not to get the Brewers yeast that is a byproduct of brewing beer. There's nothing wrong with it except the bad taste. Nutritional yeast tastes great, and adds a wonderful flavor to anything. It's especially tasty in tomato dishes and tastes good stirred into orange juice.[22]

I recommend yeast to everybody as a superfood dietary supplement. I have been asked a couple of times, "Is yeast bad?" Yes, some types of yeast are extremely problematic. We've all heard of candida, a kind of yeast that wreaks havoc on so many people, particularly women. 20 to 30 years ago, this yeast was virtually unknown. Now, it's a major health concern. The good yeast actually keeps the bad yeast from proliferating. If you are deficient in the right kind of microbes, there is nothing to fight the bad microbes. If you have bad microbes in you now, just send in reinforcements. Send in the good guys. Give your body plenty of probiotics.

One last thought on supplements. Some say supplements are not natural which is partly true. Some supplements use less than natural extraction methods while some are synthesized. It's always a good idea to get the most natural ones you can find. Some of my raw food friends believe you don't need supplements and all you need is fresh organic whole food in its natural state to be healthy. I love this idea. This is not the Garden of Eden, unfortunately, and we are exposed to a huge array of toxins and stressors. We can use all the help we can get.

One very beneficial supplement I haven't talked about enough is vitamin C. There are definitely whole books written about this one. It is probably the most famous supplement of all, and for good reason. Here's a use for it I mentioned briefly before. It's called a Vitamin C flush. All you do is get some powdered Vitamin C, pour into a glass of water, stir, and drink. You can also use capsule or tablet vitamin C. You want about the equivalent of at least 10,000 mg. This flush has a highly laxative effect, but is gentle and predictable. The Vitamin C flush also bolsters your immune system. The flush is very beneficial to do on a regular basis when you are detoxing. You should feel a lift from the process too. It's a great thing to do the night before a race or test, or any other taxing event.

Vitamin C is not stored in the body for more than a few hours, and so you should supplement throughout the day. I put powdered Vitamin C in all my drinks, except vegetable juice. I recommend you do some research on Vitamin C, to deepen your appreciation of this essential nutrient.[23] It is so essential that both carnivores and omnivores naturally produce their own. Our natural foods, unlike theirs, are full of vitamin C, so we did not evolve this ability.

As you get cleaner and healthier, you will be less and less able to handle environmental toxins. Huh? I hear you saying, "I thought everything was going to get better as I get cleaner". Yes, everything except your ability to tolerate environmental toxins. Your body will let you know immediately when it wants to be removed from an environment. Your sense of smell will become much more acute when it comes to toxins. You will be able to walk into a building that has new carpet for instance, or fresh paint, and immediately be aware that this is not somewhere your body wants to be. If you choose to stay, this feeling will go away because your body always serves your free will. You can override any message from the body. As you get cleaner and healthier, these messages become more and more clear and urgent.

I've actually become nauseous from being around fresh varnishes. Fresh paint will sometimes make me feel woozy as well. I have never been able to handle cigarette smoke very well. This aversion is one reason I never had a career in music. I am a very serious musician, but the next step for most bands is to play the clubs. I could never do this. Turns out my body was doing me a huge favor by not allowing me to play the bars. Cigarette smoke it turns out has 44 different carcinogens in it, one of which is cadmium.

Cadmium is showing itself to be one of the very worst environmental toxins. Problem is it's in so many things these days. Environmental toxins are virtually unavoidable. Unless you live in the rain forest or the wilds of Alaska, you will be exposed to them on a daily basis. Of course, we want to limit our exposure as much as possible, but the real defense is in building and maintaining a strong immune system, and embracing the blessing of being alerted by your body when you encounter toxins. Becoming more sensitive to them is actually a good thing. It can help you avoid them. Developing your nose for toxins is a byproduct of cleansing.

Some minerals you can actually get too much of. We talked about calcium, and how even when the right kind is supplied to the body, it is not well absorbed if vitamin D and magnesium are not present. I have read that zinc and selenium can be toxic if you get too much. I have experimented with high doses of both and have never reached that level. The one you really have to watch out for is iron.[24] It can build up to toxic levels easily. When this happens, your blood thickens, among other problems. There are two types of iron. Heme iron, is the one you get from red meat. Actually, I'm hoping you don't. There is also some in the dark meat of fowl. Or should we spell it foul? Heme iron was thought to be the kind that was most desirable, because it is the easiest to absorb. The kind you get from plants is not so well absorbed. New research is showing that while this is true, it is actually more desirable to get your iron from plant sources. Your body will pick up what it needs from plant sources, and no more. When it comes from animal sources, the heme iron is so well absorbed that your body cannot help but pick it up. This can cause toxic levels to accumulate. Dare I say it? This is further proof that we are not omnivores.

Just when I think this list is getting too long and I should stop, I think of something to add. Keep in mind this list is just a sampling of the superfoods that are available to age you in reverse. I just got the latest issue of Life Extension Magazine. There is an article about a seed I have been using for years— Chia. This seed has had a reputation for enhancing energy levels. The article told me several things I didn't know about Chia. It said Chia seeds have the most EFAs of any plant food. Chia is especially rich in ALA (alpha linolenic acid), which is the precursor to Omega-3. ALA, along with CLA (comjugated linolenic acid) is also known to facilitate fat loss.

The word "Chia" is Mayan for strength. The seed originates in Central America, where it has been used for centuries. It has 6 times more calcium than cow's milk—and you can actually absorb it. It is said to be a complete protein—not that it matters. I use it by soaking the seeds and making a thick milk, which I then add to other milks in small amounts. It has way too much fiber for my taste. The fiber in it is beneficial because it can keep you feeling full and not hungry for hours. The seeds, when soaked become gelatinous and can be used in recipes that call for eggs or butter.

To quote from the LEF article: "Chia has shown promise in cancer prevention. In a pre-clinical study involving breast cancer models, researchers found that dietary chia inhibited both the overall growth and the spread of cancer."

There's more: "Preclinical research suggests that chia supplementation can prevent the insulin resistance that leads to diabetes. In animals fed a sugar rich diet, chia seeds were also shown to favorably modify blood lipid changes." 'Blood lipids' include triglycerides and cholesterol. We need all the help we can get with those. Chia raises the level of HDL cholesterol. Costco has a great price on pre-packaged organic chis seeds. They have great deals on coconut water and other staples as well.

I have talked a lot in the book about what not to eat in order to age in reverse and attain a state of super health unimaginable to the average person. Since the harmful "foods" are so harmful, stopping them is a huge component—the most important part of age reversal. One of the best things about stopping them is now you have to replace them. Now the adventure begins. Learning new ways of preparing food. Experimenting with new foods, and eating a lot more of the foods that truly nourish the body.

Your excess fat melts off its own accord once you stop poisoning the body with the wrong kind of fat and too much sugar in all its many forms. I'm trying to keep this book relatively short and easy to read. I have not included many recipes because there are probably hundreds of books that deal with healthy vegan and raw recipes. There are even whole books devoted to smoothie recipes.

I would like to take a minute to make you aware of some fruits that actually incinerate fat. These are pineapple, mango, mangosteen, papaya, watermelon, and grapefruit. Strawberries also help in this regard, although they are not as potent fat burners as these other fruits.

I hope you will experiment a lot with berries of all kinds. Berries are super foods—especially the darker ones like blackberries and blueberries. We talked about tart cherries and their many health benefits. Black cherries, especially in juice form, have a wonderful laxative effect on the body. Drink a quart of black cherry juice and see what I mean. I use sweet cherries (organic of course) in some of my nut milkshakes. If you're not a member of Costco, the big bulk warehouse store, you're missing the best deals on organic frozen berries and fruits.

Berries have a substance called anthocyanin, which has been shown to have a multitude of benefits in the body, and has even been known to help reverse atherosclerosis.[25] I've even read of it being used as a cancer treatment. Elderberries and blackberries are probably the most potent source of this amazing antioxidant super substance.

I could go on and on about the wonders of fruit and vegetable super foods but this has been done very well in other books. You can also do a Google search on any food or supplement that interests you. If we include the super foods in every meal, and eat predominantly salads, vegetables, fruits, nuts, seeds, seaweed, mushrooms, onions and beans we will avail ourselves of the magic of age reversal.

If we set our intention on what we want, we will have it. We are not giving up anything! We are gaining something very few people will ever attain. Super health. I cannot begin to tell you what this is about. If I could it wouldn't do you any good anyway. You must experience it to understand. Be strong in the beginning. Set a firm intention. Use your power of volition. As you add more and more of the super foods to your diet and your life, your desire for the foods that were hastening your demise falls away. As you embrace the light, the darkness vanishes. Reach for what you want and what you don't want retreats into nothingness. What you don't want will never be a problem if you stop reaching for it. Your addictions have no hold on you unless you choose them. Free will is your salvation.

Super foods don't actually age you in reverse. Your body does. You are living in this divine instrument. You have no idea what it can do. It is powerful beyond anything you can now imagine. As you witness the body aging in reverse, you will become acquainted with its unbelievable power of regeneration. Please don't believe me. Don't believe anything. Experience is all that matters. I am very excited for you to experience age reversal. This will prove to be the most fun you have ever had. As you have this experience, you impart this experience to everyone everywhere. If you ever wanted to be a positive force for change in this world, now you have your chance. If you have ever felt powerless, you are about to feel real power. Summon the will to set your intention on what you want. It is as easy as you let it be. Keep reaching for the good stuff. All you have to do is focus on what you want, what you don't want drops out of the picture.

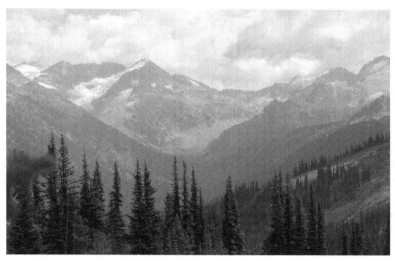

View of the glacier from Blackcomb Mountain, British Columbia

"Every tomorrow is determined by every today."

\- Paramahansa Yogananda

CONCLUSION

T his book has been a labor of love for me. Something I've dreamed about writing for many years. It has been my privilege to share with you my journey to super health and what I consider a high beyond all highs. I have a buzz that never stops. If you could feel it, if I could give you one minute to sit in this body, I guarantee you would want this drug. You would kill for this drug. Luckily, the only killing you have to do is of your addictions...stop feeding them. This lightness of being cannot even be described. I have tried, but words never do it justice, or even give you an insight on how it feels to be light and clean, how it feels to get better with each passing year. All you need to tap into this incredible energy and love of life is to stop sabotaging your body. It's easy enough to read and understand that the bad food is so much worse than you ever imagined.

The challenge is in changing your thoughts around food, in rising above your conditioning, in opening yourself to new experiences. I hear people say things like, "If I couldn't eat what I want, life would be so boring." My answer? 'Get a life'. If food is your entertainment, you're not very well entertained! If you crave a certain food, you are craving a drug effect. You are craving the taste, the tactile sensation of texture. You can have all the good taste you want in something that's healthy and will enhance your buzz.

The media is not on your side and is largely responsible for your thinking of food in very unhealthy, compulsive ways. The media seeks to induce compulsion, to make you want what they are selling at a very deep level. This has influenced your thinking much more than you know. Even if we reject these messages intellectually, they get in subliminally. I've even had people argue with me that food DOES make you happy.

They are focused on the drug effect. Drugs 'make you happy' in the same way, but the feeling is extremely temporary, and food even more so. If you take a drink or drug, you are high for a couple of hours or more. If you get your fake joy from food, the enjoyment usually lasts for 10 to 15 minutes or less. There seems to be much more bang for your buck in drugs, and they may actually do less damage to your body than the horrible foods people routinely ingest. Once you feel the real high, you won't want either.

If we can rise above our conditioning, if we can reconnect with our free will, we will truly be free. Most people are not. It takes practice. It takes bringing yourself back to your ideals. It's no good fighting against that which you don't want. All we have to do is reach for more of what we do want. I have found that when we reach for more of the good stuff, the desire for the crap goes away. Don't focus on what you are trying to quit, just reach for the good stuff. The more of the good stuff you put in, the less of the bad stuff you'll want. Soon, the desire for the crap will go away entirely.

The battle is only in the beginning. You only need willpower to make the change. Once the change is made and you feel the difference, you will not be tempted. Food and drugs promise much, but deliver so little enjoyment. If you can muster the fortitude to make these changes, you will be rewarded beyond your wildest dreams. No matter where you are physically now, you can regenerate.

If there is life in the body, there is hope. Your body wants to express its divinity. This is what homeostasis is…your body making the best of whatever you throw at it until it can no longer do so. Humans are a unique expression of nature. The human hand is said to be the most complex structure in the natural world. The colon is also unique to the human animal. As far as I know, we are the only animal where the female is receptive to mating at all times during the year. In other animals, the male is always capable of mating, but is only interested in doing so when he smells that scent. The females only emit their scent a couple of times each year or less. This makes for quite a lot of fun and drama for humans and shows one more side of our uniqueness. God truly has a sense of humor.

If we can find the fun and the joy in life, the humor in every situation, we will probably think much as God does. The spiritual Masters say the human animal is the only one that can contact God directly. They say we have come through the animal kingdom, incarnation after incarnation, to take human birth.

This is the opportunity we have been given. Your body is like a lump of clay you can mold in any way you see fit. It is your choice whether you make something beautiful, something hideous, or something in between. It is yours to do with what you will. What will you make of your body? Will you work with it, listening to what it tells you? Will you use it for a source of cheap entertainment, heedless to its continued cries for mercy? Once you start to listen to your body, it will always let you know if what you are doing is working.

Just be sure as you are making these changes, the body is not detoxifying too quickly and giving you false readings. Remember, just by not eating the heavy foods that were attacking it puts the body into cleanse mode. You must keep pace with this cleansing. You must continue to support the cleansing process through enemas, herbs, and patience. If you cannot bring yourself to try enemas and colonics, at least use some herbal laxatives like aloe or cascara sagrada. There are many good herbal laxative formulations. Any health food store will have something to help you eliminate more solid waste, which you must do during this cleansing process. If you change your diet for the better and feel worse, it is due to elimination. More specifically, you are not keeping pace with elimination.

You don't need to gradually eliminate these foods from your diet, but that may be what happens, due to a lack of willpower. That is fine. No worries. However long it takes to weed these enemies to your health out of your life forever is time well spent. Remember, the longer you go between times of weakness and caving in to your desires to eat crap, the more you will feel the adverse effect when you do. This helps you stay strong because you know you're going to pay if you eat the junk. Just enjoy the process. Take it easy on yourself.

This is all a lot of fun. If you fall off the wagon, just jump back on. It will probably help if you can find someone who's doing this at the same time. You can support each other. I was alone in this process. As you start to feel the difference, you will have all the motivation you need. When you get to the other side of this process, and are free, you will find it hard to believe you ever ate that crap. You will wonder how people can be walking around while eating that stuff on a daily basis. You will be moved to try to help them. You will already be doing so just by doing it yourself.

We influence each other on the telepathic and subliminal level. You will help everyone to a better life as you achieve one yourself. You will become part of the solution. You will help humankind to walk more gently upon this earth. You will help to save our species from certain extinction. If we go on the way we are, our species is not sustainable. We have become like a parasite on this earth. This time the parasite cannot destroy its host. It can only destroy itself and take many other species with it.

It's been said that the production of meat is the single biggest environmental hazard we generate. It's hard to believe meat production could be worse than nuclear power and weapons, but as far as survival of our species goes, it may be true.

The suffering we visit on our fellow creatures will, and indeed, has come back to haunt us. Animals have souls just as we do, though not at the same state of evolution. Stopping our exploitation and cruelty to animals will go a long way toward restoring our humanity. Man's inhumanity to man is at the heart of our troubles. As we regain our health by stopping the consumption of meat, dairy and eggs, we stop the destruction of compassion.

If you had to kill these animals yourself, you would probably never eat their meat. If you had to clean their dead bodies, getting blood all over your hands, you would most certainly not want to eat their muscle tissue or internal organs.

I haven't said much about eggs, but if you look at a raw egg, the white part looks like snot. Indeed, eggs are highly mucous forming. If you have to eat eggs, throw away the white part and eat the yolk, but better not to eat them at all. A quote from the Journal of the American Medical Association may help motivate you to give them up: "Women who ate eggs three or more days each week had a three times greater risk of fatal ovarian cancer than did women who ate eggs less than one day per week." Imagine what would happen to your cancer risk if you ate none.

As you raise your vibration by changing your diet, you will not want to consume congealed chicken embryos. As you become more attuned to your body, you will not want to put anything in it to gum up the works. As you develop more self-control, you will find this blessing spills over into every aspect of your life. As I have said before, you will become calm and peaceful. Eventually, virtually nothing will make you mad.

There are many other benefits of this lifestyle. Your ability to enjoy heat and cold will be enhanced dramatically. I have found as I get cleaner and healthier, I can stand extreme heat so much better than I ever could before. I rather like cold weather, but have never really enjoyed hot weather. I still don't so much, but heat doesn't bother me as it used to.

As you get cleaner, you may feel it can't get any better. You wonder how you could feel any better than you do. You can't imagine anything more wonderful than the way you feel. Yet, it gets better and better all the time. There is no end. Well, I guess there is, but who cares? In the moment, you will continue to feel more and more amazing.

This is my experience. No one can tell me age reversal is not possible. I live it. I experience it on a daily basis. I hope you will have this experience too. I know you can if you will allow yourself the experience.

Conditioning drops away. Limitations cease to exist. Limitations are self-imposed. If you stop feeding them, they will go away. We need not seek enlightenment, we have it already. We only need to stop cherishing beliefs. Remember belief counts for nothing. Experience is all that matters. Whether something is true or not cannot be known by reading something or having someone tell you something. You will find out the truth in any statement by trying and experiencing. Please don't take my word for any of this. If any of this information resonates with you, try it out and see if it is real. Relax and enjoy the ride. Life is about to become a lot more fun.

RECIPE FOR NUT AND SEED MILKS

1. Soak your nuts or seeds. Some nuts do not absorb water and do not need to be soaked. Some of these include pine nuts, Brazil nuts, and macadamia nuts. Any nut or seed that will absorb water should be soaked, except for cashews which are so soft they do not need to be soaked but can be.
2. Include the soak water in the nut milk or drink separately or use in recipes. If any nut turns the soak water red or brown, that soak water should be discarded. Nuts that turn the soak water red include walnuts, pecans, and hazelnuts. Put your soaked nuts into your blender. If you have not included the soak water, add water sufficient to liquefy your nuts– about a 1 to 1 ratio. We want to use as little water as possible to get maximum agitation.
3. Turn the blender on set on a low speed setting, with the high/low setting set on low. This keeps your nuts from being thrown in pieces to the sides of the blender. Dial the speed setting up to 10, and then flip the high/low switch to high. Blend longer than you probably think is necessary (2-3 minutes). If you hear the blender start to run at a higher pitch, it means you need to add water. Sometimes the blending process uses up the water and you need to add more. Remove the plug in the hole in the lid and pour some water in, no need to stop the machine. Most blenders like the Vita mix have a handy hole in the lid for this purpose. Remove the plug and add just enough water so that the machine starts blending again.

After you have completed the blending process, add your fruit and blend starting once again with a low speed and progressing to high. Always get in the habit of flipping the high/low switch to low and dialing the speed setting back down to 3 or so. When you turn the blender on again set on the high setting it can be very loud and startle you. If you are making just the milk without fruit, add water or coconut water to the consistency desired, and mix on a low setting. Always mix on a low setting to avoid bubbles forming on the top of your milk. If you have made a large amount for storage later, pour off into a container (preferably Glass) what you are not using now, store in the refrigerator. It will keep for at least a week refrigerated.

HOW TO DO ENEMAS

Good quality enema bags are hard to come by. I have found a very good quality one made by a company called Cara Inc. They call it a "Water Bottle Combination". I got mine at a pharmacy. This particular pharmacy is the only place in Atlanta I have found to buy this. I will therefore include their address; 333 Strawberry Field Rd., Warwick, RI 02886. This is a very high quality rig, which can also be used as a hot water bottle.

So here's a little step-by-step on how to do your first internal cleanse. The bag holds a little less than 2 quarts. Try a quart for your first one. Always use filtered or distilled water. Heat the water to body (tepid) temperature in anything but the hottest weather.

1. Put as much water in the bag as you desire. Screw the cap with the hose attached into the bag. Turn the bag upside down and let some of the water out to purge the air from the bag. The bag comes with a clamp to stop the water coming out or to slow the flow. I find it easier to dispense with the clamp and

use my fingers. You can also bend the hose over on itself and pinch to stop the flow completely while you insert the rectal attachment.

2. Stopping the flow of water by pinching the tube in whichever way you find easiest, insert the rectal attachment. Holding the rectal attachment in with one hand, hang the bag somewhere around four to five feet off the floor. The higher you hang the bag the faster the water will flow unless the hose is pinched.

3. Holding the rectal attachment in, drop down on to one knee and one elbow. You can drop down to two knees. I find it easiest to hold the rectal tube with my left hand while I drop down to my right forearm and elbow and right knee, with my left ball of the foot on the floor.

4. Allow the water to flow in; controlling the speed it flows in by pinching the hose or allowing it to run full speed. If it feels like it's going too fast, don't hesitate to pinch the hose and stop it completely. This feeling will pass and you will be able to finish the fill. Relax. Breathe.

5. When you are done filling wash the rectal tube, empty whatever water may be left in the bag, and hang it upside down to dry. Store your hose, after running some water through it, in a straight position. I use a piece of wire to hang it on a towel bar. The bag and the hose must be hung so they can drain and dry completely. I use a denture-cleaning tablet every now and then to keep the bag completely clean.

As you are more practiced doing enemas you may want to experiment with holding the water longer, letting it absorb more toxins. For now just go to the toilet and let it out. Be sure you're sitting completely down on the toilet before you let fly. (Don't ask me how I know this) You can do as many enemas as you want. The more the better while you are detoxing. Enjoy learning this new skill. Enjoy especially the feeling of lightness after this cleanse. Work toward using the whole bag; somewhere close to 2 quarts, every time.

Be assured this is the best way to assist your body in getting rid of toxins. Remember, detoxing is a two-stage process. When you stop eating the junk the toxins are mobilized—taken out of suspension and put into circulation. Your job is to facilitate elimination. You don't want them circulating any longer than necessary. This new skill will support the detoxing process better than anything I know of. There is absolutely no danger in doing this (other than making a mess). Just kidding. I have never made a mess in 40 years of doing enemas, other than just a little overspray on the back of the toilet. Have fun.

RECIPE FOR PROBIOTIC SAUERKRAUT WATER, aka REJUVELAC

1. Finely chop, food process, or blend veggies. Use pulp from juicing if you have it.
2. Put veggies in a gallon jar. I use one that does not "neck down". The kind that looks like an old-fashioned candy jar is the best. The glass lid on these is the same diameter as the jar. I got mine at Walmart.
3. Fill the jar about a third of the way up with the veggies. Add water, leaving an inch or so of "headspace", or room at the top below the lid.

247

4. Put the lid on and keep out of sunlight to preserve the nutritional content of the veggies. Light degrades nutrients, which is why vitamins are sold in dark glass bottles.
5. Let sit for at least 24 hrs. if the room is warm. If the room is not sufficiently warm the wild culture will not form. Taste it to see if it has "made". I use a straw to reach to the liquid portion to sample it.(the pulp rises to the top) If mold appears on top you will know it is ready. Scrape off the mold. The drink will be fine.
6. Strain through a coarse strainer. I use a large strainer put into a gallon pitcher. Use a large spoon to press the pulp against the strainer. Use the pulp as compost or discard. I throw it on my yard grass. Strain through a fine strainer into another pitcher. Pour the strained drink into a glass bottle or jar, cap and refrigerate. It keeps for weeks refrigerated.

NOTES

INTRODUCTION

[1] Fung TT, Hu FB, Hankinson SE, Willet WC, Holmes MD. Low carbohydrate diets, dietary approaches to stop hypertension and the risk of postmenopausal breast cancer. George Roth PhD, Gero Science Inc. Pylesville, Maryland National Institute on Aging (NIA)

[2] Samskaras– a Sanskrit word referring to past life tendencies. This includes talents and adversions.
Paramhansa Yogananda—Autobiography of a Yogi
Eckart Tolle—The Power of Now
Robert Adams—Happiness this Moment

[3] Prana– a Sanskrit word referring to the life force energy that we live on. Pranayamas are exercises developed in ancient India to control (yama) the life force.

DEADLY DAIRY

[1] Harris W, The scientific basis of vegetarianism, Less grains more greens, Hawaii Health Publishers
Furhman J, Eat to Live pp 108

[2] Robbins, diet for a new America, pp 97
Grant WB, Milk and other influences on coronary heart disease

[3] Liechtenstein AH, Ausman LM, Jalbert SM, Shaefer EJ, Effects of different forms of dietary hydrogenated fats on serum lipoprotein cholesterol levels– New England Journal of Medicine

[4] New SA, Robbins SP, Campbell MA, et al. dietary influences on bone mass and bone metabolism: further

evidence of a positive link between fruit and vegetable consumption and bone health? American Journal of clinical nutrition

5   Browner WS et al, Non trauma mortality in elderly women with low bone mineral density. Study of Osteoporotic Fractures Research group, Lancet

Grant WB, Milk and other influences on coronary heart disease, Alternative Medical Review

Segall JJ, epidemiological evidence for the link between dietary lactose and antherosclerosis. Glycation hypothesis of antherosclerosis

6   Knapen MHK et. al. effect of vitamin K supplementation on circulating osteocalcin and urinary calcium excretion

Olson RE, The function and metabolism of vitamin K

Vervoort LM et.al. The potent antioxidant activity of the vitamin K cycle in microsomal lipid peroxidation

7   Bosetti C, Tzonou A, Lagiou P, et.al. Fraction of prostate cancer attributed to diet in Athens Greece. European Journal of Cancer Prevention

Chan JM, Stampfer MJ, Ma J, et.al. Dairy products, calcium and prostate cancer risk positions health study

Robbins J, Diet for a New America pp 70

8   Kulvanaskas V, Survival into the 21st Century

9   Massey LK, Dietary animal and plant protein in human bone health: a whole foods approach. Journal of Nutrition

Fuhrman J, Eat to Live, pp 140

10   Fuhrman J, Eat to Live, pp 108

US Environmental Protection Agency. National Center for Environmental Assessment.

11   Welch AA, Mulligan A, Bingham SA, et.al. Urine pH is an indicator of dietary acid-base load. Results from the European perspective investigation into Cancer and nutrition

12 Dan Hammer, www.agingnomore.com
13 Wigmore Ann, Be Your Own Doctor.
14 Mercola.com
15 About.comHealth benefits of basil
    Lifescript.com/Health
16 Enwikipedia.org/wk/casomorphine
    Ownahealthyheart.com
    Gomestic.com-
    cheezehasalittleknownsecret/consumersbeware

MEAT: DEATH IN, DEATH OUT

1   Yoav Gilad Ph.D, Associate professor of human genetics,
    University of Chacago
    Audrey L. Mammon MD Ph.D, Johns Hopkins
    American Society of Human Genetics
2   Dr. Norman Walker, Become Younger
    Kulvanaskas V, Survival into the 21st Century
    Fuhrman J MD, The End of Dieting
3   www.cancer.org
4   answers.yahoo.com/question index
    www.nature.com/scitable/topicpage/themysteryofvitaminc
    www.fruitliving.com
    HappySexyHealthy.net
    www.davidicke.com/humansvscarnivores
5   Tucker KL, Osteoporosis prevention and nutrition
    Fuhrman J, Eat to Live, pp 103-04
6   Fuhrman J, Eat to Live, pp 125
7   www.ejnet.org/bgh/nogood.html
    www.livestrong.com>hormoneconditions
    www.ehow.com
    www.breastcancerfund.org/bovinegrowthhormone.html
8   Robbins J, Diet for a New America, pp 316

9   guardian/v.com
    www.gmocompass.org
    www.dairyherd.com/topics/genetically-modified-
    organisims-o
10 Barnard MD, Nicholson A, Howard JL, The medical costs
    attributed to meat consumption
    Fuhrman J, Eat to Live, pp 97
11 www.webmd.com
    www.sciencedaily.com
    www.endocrinewatch.com
12 Virtanen JK, Mozafferian D, Chiuve SE, Rimm EB, Fish
    consumption and risk of major chronic disease in men
    Black JJ, Bauman PC, Carcinogens and cancers in
    freshwater fishes
13 Fuhrman J, Eat to Live, pp 130
14 www.wisegeekhealth.com/whataresuperbacteria.htm
    www.feelgoodagain.com/supergerms.htm
15 www.codexalementarius.org This is the official website. It
    will make CODEX sound like a good thing. Further
    research is needed to get to the truth about what it takes
    away in terms of our health freedom
16 www.webmd.com
    www.rarediseasesabout.com
    www.endocrinehealth.com
    Kick R, Everything You Know Is Wrong, pp 89
17 environment.nationalgeographic/enviornmentalphotos-
    rivers-run-dry
    Centerpunch.org/why-the-colorado-river-doesn't-meet-
    the-sea

PROTEIN—HOW MUCH IS TOO MUCH?

[1] www.rawfoodexplaned.com/proteins/complete-proteins.html
Some websites are still talking how to make a complete protein by combining foods—the myth is anything but dead
[2] www.madcowboy.com
omhats.com/oprah-sued-by-beef-association
[3] https://answers.yahoo.com
www.muscleforlife.com Here's one site of many that says the fact that one can only absorb 30 gr. of protein at a time is a myth. I invite you to do your own research—especially by trying eating less, then seeing how you feel eating more. This is the REAL test.
[4] www.muscleandfitnesstips.org
Forumbodybuilding.com
www.muscleandstrength.com
[5] Fuhrman J, Eat to Live, pp 76-77
www.reuters.com
There are several other sites talking about how the USDA buys surplus milk to keep the price artificially high. Some mention the programs it donated all this milk and cheese to.

WHEAT IS NO TREAT

[1] Jarvi AF, Karlsteom BE, Grandfeldt YE, et.al. The influence of food structure in postprandial metabolism in patients with non-insulin resistant diabetes. American Journal of Clinical Nutrition 1995 Apr.
Davis W, Wheat Belly, pp 32-36
[2] Juntunen KS, Niskanin LK, Liukkonen KH, et.al. Postprandial glucose, insulin and incretin responses to grain products in healthy subjects. American Journal of Clinical Nutrition 202 Feb.

[3] Jenkins DJH, Wolever TM, Taylor RH, et.al. Glycemic index of foods: a physiological basis for carbohydrate exchange. American Journal of Clinical Nutrition 1981 Mar.

[4] www.mayoclinic.org/diseases-conditions/medibolic-syndrome
www.emedicinehealth.com/thyroid+metabolism
www.drweil.com/Medibolic-Syndrome.html

[5] thepaleodiet.com
ultimatepaleoguide.com
www.atkins.com
lowcarbdiets.about.com

[6] brainoverbinge.blogspot.com
www.marksdailyapple.com

[7] www.cbsnews.com/statins-may-lower-teestosterone-libido
www.eyce/male.com/statins...Testosterone-production
douglasreport.com2010/05/19/statins lower-testosterone

[8] Fogel S, Life Extension Magazine, July 2013
Sasaki M, Joh T, Koikeda S, et.al. A novel strategy in production of oligosaccrides in digestive tract: prevention of postprandial hyperglycemia and hyperinsulinemia. Journal of Biochemical Nutrition 2007 Nov.

[9] Bjornholt NV, Erikssen G, Aaser E, et.al. Fasting blood glucose: An underestimated risk factor for cardiovascular death. Results from a 22 year study. Diabetes Care 1999

[10] www.stevia.com
www.familydoctor.org

[11] www.medicinenet.com
www.sweetpoison.com
articalsmercola.com/10/13/artificial-sweetners-more-dangerous
www.globalhealing center.com

[12] www.glycemicedge.com
www.myfit.ca/glycemic-indexasp

Note: some charts show different numbers for a given food. This is no problem for comparison purposes. It doesn't really matter if bread is 88, or as some charts say, 97. 88 is very high indeed.

[13] www.cbsnews.com/news/obese-kids-tend-to-have-metabolic-syndrome
Kidshealth.org/teen/diseases

[14] Davis W, Wheat Belly, pp 123-129

[15] About.com/WhatFoodsIsGlutenIn

[16] www.celiac.com
www.healthgrade.com>CeliacDisease

NO JOY IN SOY

[1] Daniel K, The Whole Soy Story, pp 166-169

[2] Daniel K, The Whole Soy Story, pp 27-29

[3] www.gmofoods.com
naturalscociety.com/top-10-worst-gmo-foods-list

[4] www.saynotogmo.org
www.csa.com/discoveryguides/gmofood/overview.php
www.wikinow.com>...>NutritionalLifestyleEating

[5] www.anci.cornell.edu/plants/toxicagents/aflotoxin.html

[6] www.sourcewatch.org/index-php/Roundup-Ready

[7] Daniel K, The Whole Soy Story, pp 162-163

[8] www.coppertoxic.com
www.holistic-back-relief.com/coppertoxicity.html
www.diagnose-me/symptoms-of/copper-toxicity.html

[9] HealthyReply.com/ZincDeficiencySign
www.rightdiagnosis.com>Diseases>zincdeficiency

[10] Daniel K, The Whole Soy Story, pp 122-128

[11] www.fearlessfatloss.com/What-is-the-ingredient-natural-flavor
goaskalice.columbia.edu>...>Nutrition

12   Daniel K, The Whole Soy Story, pp 128-130
13   Emedicine.medscape.com/article1174981
14   Daniel K, The Whole Soy Story, pp 236-239
15   Daniel K, The Whole Soy Story, pp 175-176
16   Daniel K, The Whole Soy Story, pp 142-143, 213-222
17   Daniel K, The Whole Soy Story, pp 239-243
18   Daniel K, The Whole Soy Story, pp 230, 236
19   www.lowoxalate.info
     alwayswellwithin.com/2010/04/27/high-oxalate-foods-can-trigger
20   Daniel K, The Whole Soy Story, pp 295-393
21   Brownstein D, Overcoming Thyroid Disorders
     Brownstein D, Iodine Why You Need It
     www.thyroid.org
     www.emedicinehealth.com>thyroid

SPIRITUALITY AND AGE-REVERSAL

1   Icke D, Alice in Wonderland and the World Trade Center Disaster
2   www.PolymyosisTreatment.com
3   www.drugwatch.com/crestor/side-effects
4   Perlmutter D, Grain Brain, pp 131
5   Perlmutter D, Grain Brain, pp 150-153
6   www.ncbi.nlm.nib.gov/pubmed/20814420
7   www.quizlet.com/subject/term%3Ablood%20supply
     www.wisegeek.com/how-much-oxygen-and-calories-does-the-brain-need
8   www.2knowmyself.com/subconscious-mind
9   Adams R, Silence of the Heart

MUSCLE IS YOUTH

[1] https://uk.answers.yahoo.com/questions/index?qid =20080402043405AAIK5yS
wwwanswers.com>Categories>Health>Fitness>Exercise
[2] www.goodfats.pamlotella.com
[3] Life Extension Magazine, April 2013, How Antherosclerosis Develops in Aging Humans
[4] Robbins J, Diet for a New America, pp 248-273
[5] Davis D, Disconnect book
[6] www. Apoptosis.com
biologyabout.com>Cell Biology>CellularProcesses
[7] www.glutathionediseasecare.com-aceytlcystine

PROBIOTICS

[1] Shoemaker R, Mold Warriors book, www.survivingmold.com

FOOD COMBINING

[1] www.fitday.com>Home>Nutrition>Healthy Eating
articlesmercola.com/.../05probiotics...your-gut-is-your-immune-system.aspx
[2] www.acidreflux.com
www.medicinenet.com>...>heartburn
[3] Walker N, Become Younger
Kulvinaskas V, Survival into the 21st Century
[4] Fuhrman J, Eat to Live
[5] Life Extension Magazine, April 2013, Astaxanthin Provides Broad Spectrum Protection
[6] Wwwepa.gov>climatechange>emissions>overview
[7] www.nytimes.com/2000/04/20/us/2-fiber-studies-find-no-benefit-for

www.eurekalert.org/pub-releases/2013-10

[8] Taubes G, Good Calories Bad Calories pp122-135

[9] Chemistry about.com>...>Food&Cooking Chemistry

ATHEROSCLEROSIS

[1] Life Extension Magazine, November 2014, Enhance Endothelial Health—How Pomegranate Protects against antherosclerosis

[2] www.howtoreducebadcholesterol.com
www.sharecare.com>ImproveYourCholesterol

[3] www.webmd.com>cholesterol&trigliceridesguide

[4] www.drweil.com/Elevated-Homosystiene

[5] www.mayoclinic.org/cholesterol/in-depth/trans-fat

[6] Daniel K, The Whole Soy Story, pp 232-336

[7] Life Extension Magazine, Nov. 2014 pp 57

[8] Life Extension Magazine, June 2013 Anti-inflammatory properties of Tart Cherry

[9] Circ.ahajournals.org/content/109/23

[10] www.exibithealth.com/general-health/healthbenefitsofboswella
www.superfoods-scientificresearch.com/boswella-benefits.html

[11] www.medicalnewstoday.com?articiles/248423

[12] Pottenger F, Pottenger's Cats
www.enzyme-facts.com/francispottenger

[13] Archive.crohn.ie/primer/inflresp.htm

[14] www.mayoclinic.org/tests-procedures-reactive-protein

[15] HealthyReply.comVitaminDDeficiency
www.naturalnews.com/035089

[16] Emedicine.medscape.com/article/2085501

[17] www.wisegeek.com/what-is-fibrinogen

18 www.medicinenet.com>...>highbloodpressurehypertansion index
19 Cholesterolabout.com.typesofcholesterol
    Articals.mercola.com.../05/dr-robert-rowan-part2
20 Wikihow.com>...>Food and Entertaining>FoodPreparation
21 Sleepless In America, National Geographic Channel

WATER

1 ezineaeticles.com>HealthandFitness>EnviornmentalIssues
   philforhumanity.com/Bottledwaterhtml
2 www.worldometers.info/world-population
   www.census.gov>...>Data>InternationalDataBase
3 Murad H, The Water Secret
4 https://answers.yahoo.com/question/index?qid
   =2008072674335AAHe1Ao

JUICING AND NUT MILKS

1 www.inteliReview.com
   www.fernsnutrition.com/Juicer-types.htm
2 www.tribestlife.com
3 Vitamix.com
4 About.com/TypesofCalcium
5 Fuhrman J, Eat to Live, pp 103-104
   Blog.seattlepi.com/naturalnotes/2009/09/01/magnesium-
   and-calcium
6 Fuhrman J, Eat to Live, pp 106-111
7 jerrysnuthouse.com/why-you-should-be-eating-raw-nuts
   articles.mercola.com/sites/articles/archive/2012/03/29/
   raw-nuts
8 www.muscleandstrength.com>Articles>suppliments
9 Ask.com/WhatisMacaRootFor
   www.herbal-supplement-resorce.com/Maca-root.html

GOT AMPK?

[1] Life Extension Magazine, Winter 2014, Special Edition

DETOXIFICATION

[1] articles.mercola.com/sites/articles/archive/2012/09/24/how-sugar
www.bodybuilding.com...>FoodandRecipes>sugar-sweetners
medicosmosmle.blogspot.com/feeds/posts/default
www.researchportal.be/en/projects/browse.html?page=168
[2] health-a lot.com/AlcoholDetox
[3] www.shping.net/hydrosan.php
[4] www.buzzle.com/articles/mercury-poisoning-from-fish.html
www.medicinenet.com/mercuryarticle
[5] thefoodevolution.com/natural-remedies-for-radiation-exposure
[6] en.wikipedia.org/wiki/List-of-carcinogens-in-cigarette-smoke
jnci.oxfordjournals.org>Volume91Issue14
www.mysmokeless.com/carcinogens-in-cigarette-smoke
[7] https://www.detoxtheworld.com/tag/menstruation
www.beautifulonraw.com/.../raw-foods-and-menstruation
www.ehow.com>...>AlternativeMedicine>Fasting&Cleansing
[8] Hippocratesinst.org
[9] Walker N, Become Younger
[10] enWikipedia.org/S-Adenosyl-methionine
[11] vactruth.com2010/07/23/fact.vaccines-have-never-eradicated
www.historyofvaccines.org/content/articles/disease/eradication

12 www.immunizationinfo.org/thinerosal/mercury-vaccines
www.healingarts.org/children/vaccines/mercury.html
www.forbes.com/sites/emilywillingham/2014/02/22/is-the-cdc-hiding
13 Rogers S, Detoxify or Die, pp141-148
14 Cott A, Fasting as a Way of Life
www.fitnessthroughfasting.com
www.quickfasting.com/fasting

AGEs THAT ARE AGING YOU

1 Davis W, Wheat Belly, pp 133-139
2 Healthmad.com/nutrition/why-fried-food-causes-cancer
3 www.lef.org/magazine/2011/1/Carnosine-Exceedingexpectations
4 Davis W, Wheat Belly, pp 140-143
5 www.ncbi.nib.gov.JournalLists>AmJNephrol
www.nibi.nlm.gov/pubmed/217789583
6 Davis W, Wheat Belly, pp 33-35
7 The Truth About Exercise, PBS
8 www.lef.org/magazine/2008/4/Aging-And-Glycation
9 Peaktestosterone.com/Advanced-Glycation-End-Products
10 Innovitaresearch.org/news/06042501.html
Medical.dictionary.thefreedictionary.com/lipofuscin

SUPER FOODS & SUPPLEMENTS

1 Life Extension Magazine, Aug. 2013, New Studies Validate Efficacy of Vitamin D
Life Extension Magazine, June, 2013, Vitamin D Slows Parkinson's Progression
Life Extension Magazine, July 2014, Vitamin D Slashes Breast Cancer Mortality
2 Journey of Man, National Geographic Channel

[3] Life Extension Magazine, Aug. 2014, Fight Immune Decline With Reishi

[4] www.mushroom-appreciation.com/maitake-mushroom.html
www.healthcastle.com>CookingSmart
www.herblist.net/maitake.html

[5] www.burzynskiclinic.com

[6] www.antioxidants-for-health-anlongevity.com/chlorellaandspirolina

[7] www.sunchlorellausa.com/what-is-chlorella

[8] Brownstein D, Overcoming Thyroid Disorders

[9] fucoidanfacts.com
www.ehow.com/facts/501129/benefits-fucoidan.html

[10] www.vitamins-nutrition.org/vitamins/zinc.html
www.poliquingroup.com/../Article/1812/top-10-benefits-of-zinc

[11] www.herbalwisdom.com/herb-rhodiola.html
www.drwiel.com/drw/u/QAA400399/Rhodiola-for-what-ails-you.html

[12] About.com/HawthornHerbBenefits
www.herbalwisdom.com/herb/hawthorn-berry.html

[13] Science Daily, Cons of regular low-dose aspirin use to stave off serious illness

[14] www.ubiquinol.org
witakerhealthfreedom.com/2012/03/..be-warned-of-statin-drug-dangers

[15] Curcumin-turmeric.com
www.webmd.com/.../lifestyle-guide-suppliment-guide-turmeric

[16] Altmedicine.about.com.herbsandherbalmedicine>ephedra

[17] www.herbal-treatment-remidies.com/White-willow-bark.html
Ask.com/WillowBarkBenefits

[18] Life Extension Magazine, May 2005, DHEA Improves Vascular Health
Life Extension Magazine, Feb. 2002, DHEA Improves Postmenopausal Health
Life Extension Magazine, Oct. 2001, DHEA Reilieves Aathma
[19] www.naturalnews.com/030899-vitamin_E_brain
[20] Life Extension Magazine, Aug. 2014, Little Known Benefits of Tocotrenols
[21] www.tropicaltraditions.com/palmoil
WholeHealth.com/Red-Palm-oil
[22] www.mindbodygreen.com/why-im-obsessed-with-nutritional-yeast
[23] www.healthdiaries.com>EatThis!
About.com/VitaminCBenefits
[24] Drhoffman.com/article/iron-deficiency-and-toxicity-3
[25] www.raysahelian.com/anthocyanins.html
Life Extension Magazine, March 2000, How Berries Slow Brain Aging
Life Extension Magazine, April 2009, Berry Compounds Protect Aging Brains